Problems in Anesthesiology:

Approach to Diagnosis

Problems in Anesthesiology:
Approach to Diagnosis

Roberta E. Galford, M.D.
Staff Anesthesiologist
Grant Medical Center
Columbus, Ohio

Foreword by
Thomas W. Feeley, M.D.
Professor of Anesthesia, Stanford University
School of Medicine, Stanford, California

Little, Brown and Company
Boston/Toronto/London

Library of Congress Cataloging-in-Publication Data

Galford, Roberta E.
    Problems in anesthesiology : approach to diagnosis / Roberta
E. Galford : foreword by Thomas W. Feeley.—1st ed.
        p.   cm.
    Includes bibliographical references and index.
    ISBN 0-316-30289-9
    1. Anesthesia—Complications—Handbooks, manuals, etc.
2. Surgery—Complications—Handbooks, manuals, etc.
3.   Diagnosis, Differential—Handbooks, manuals, etc.   I. Title.
    [DNLM: 1. Anesthesia—handbooks.   2. Diagnosis,
Differential—handbooks,   3. Intraoperative Complications—
diagnosis—handbooks,   4. Postoperative Complications—
diagnosis—handbooks.   WO 231 G155p.]
    RD82.5.G35   1992
    617.9′6041—dc20
    DNLM/DLC
    for Library of Congress   92-10310
                                                                    CIP

Printed in the United States of America

RRD-VA

To Alexis for her patience and understanding
and
To Mom and Dad for their guidance
and support throughout the years

Contents

Foreword

Not too many years ago, the majority of textbooks dealing with anesthesiology were written abroad. Today, the number and variety of textbooks in anesthesiology coming from authors within the United States are tremendous. The current student of anesthesiology has several major American textbooks to choose from, as well as numerous textbooks dealing with specialized aspects of the practice of anesthesiology. Most are very good but follow a rather standard textbook format. It is therefore refreshing to find authors who are willing to experiment with new methods of writing textbooks in anesthesiology. In *Problems in Anesthesiology*, Roberta Galford has used a new format with great success.

The practice of anesthesiology is often quite routine and most of us appreciate the case that is uncomplicated and routine. Nevertheless, the real challenge is when the anesthesiologist is faced with a difficult problem, with a patient who demands immediate attention. Outstanding anesthesiologists are recognized as such, based on how they react to problems thrown their way.

Problems in Anesthesiology approaches our field from the perspective of the problems we must manage. It begins by dealing with acute respiratory problems and the first of those is hypoxia—the common denominator of many unsatisfactory outcomes of administering anesthesia. The problems are presented in a clear, crisp, and concise fashion, with a definition, an outline of possible etiologies, and a bottom-line type of discussion that presents all of the issues without wasting words. Each problem is followed by several references dealing with the topic in general terms rather than providing evidence for small points. The net result is a very readable book that will be appreciated by students, residents, anesthesiologists preparing for the Board examination, and practicing anesthesiologists.

While the problem-oriented approach is hardly new to medicine, *Problems in Anesthesiology* is a new way of presenting the field of anesthesiology to physicians. This book is a unique and outstanding contribution to the literature of American anesthesiology.

Thomas W. Feeley, M.D.

Preface

Several years ago, during my anesthesia residency, a junior attending told me that the one thing I must do to prepare for the oral boards was to compile a list of differential diagnoses for common problems encountered in the operating room. As I collected causes of various disorders, it became obvious that there was no single reference source available. I found this absence remarkable since anesthetists run through a mental checklist of possible reasons for a particular physiologic disturbance many times each day.

Therefore, I decided that a differential diagnosis book on anesthesia was needed. I wanted it to have practical application for many levels of skill and experience, from the novice to the senior attending, either in practice or in preparation for board examinations. Two caveats, however, must be mentioned. First, this text is not intended to be a "cookbook" but a reminder of the many factors that can lead to a particular clinical problem. Second, a book of this type can never be complete, as new causes of problems will continue to be discovered and reported.

Several people deserve my special thanks. Dr. Raeford Brown helped greatly in starting this project. Susan Pioli of Little, Brown provided invaluable guidance and assistance. Drs. Ted Heyneker, Timothy Harwood, Hillel Kashtan, and Daniel Kennedy did an admirable job as contributing authors. Last, but not least, Faith McLellan and the editorial staff of the Department of Anesthesia at the Bowman Gray School of Medicine of Wake Forest University spent countless hours reviewing and revising this work.

R.E.G.

Contributing Authors

Raeford E. Brown, Jr., M.D.
Associate Professor, Anesthesia and Pediatrics, University of Arkansas College of Medicine; Chief, Division of Pediatric Anesthesia, Arkansas Children's Hospital, Little Rock, Arkansas

Roberta E. Galford, M.D.
Staff Anesthesiologist, Grant Medical Center, Columbus, Ohio

Timothy N. Harwood, M.D.
Instructor, Department of Anesthesia, Bowman Gray School of Medicine of Wake Forest University; Attending Physician, North Carolina Baptist Hospitals, Winston-Salem, North Carolina

Theodore J. Heyneker, M.D.
Assistant Professor, Department of Anesthesia, Bowman Gray School of Medicine of Wake Forest University; Attending Physician, North Carolina Baptist Hospitals, Winston-Salem, North Carolina

Hillel I. Kashtan, M.D.
Assistant Professor, Department of Anesthesia, Bowman Gray School of Medicine of Wake Forest University; Attending Physician, North Carolina Baptist Hospitals, Winston-Salem, North Carolina

Daniel J. Kennedy, M.D.
Resident, Department of Anesthesia, Bowman Gray School of Medicine of Wake Forest University and North Carolina Baptist Hospitals, Winston-Salem, North Carolina

I
Respiratory

1
Hypoxia/Hypoxemia

DEFINITION

Hypoxia is defined as inadequate tissue oxygenation. This term is often used interchangeably with hypoxemia, which means deficient oxygen tension (PaO_2) in the arterial blood. Tissue oxygenation is dependent on oxygen transport to the tissues and oxygen utilization by the tissues; oxygen transport is the product of cardiac output (C.O.) and arterial oxygen content (CaO_2). Causes of hypoxia can be divided into three major categories: (1) ischemic hypoxia, due to inadequate tissue perfusion, (2) hypoxemic hypoxia, due to inadequate oxygen content, and (3) toxic hypoxia, due to impaired oxygen utilization. The oxygen content can be lowered by three mechanisms: (1) reduced arterial oxygen tension (PaO_2)—hypoxic hypoxemia, (2) decreased hemoglobin—anemic hypoxemia, and (3) altered hemoglobin-oxygen binding (SaO_2)—toxic hypoxemia.

ETIOLOGY

   I. Ischemic hypoxia
      A. Decreased cardiac output
      B. Atherosclerotic vascular disease
  II. Hypoxemic hypoxia
      A. Hypoxic hypoxemia
         1. Low inspired oxygen tension (FiO_2) (flowmeter error, decreased oxygen tension)
         2. Reduced alveolar oxygen tension (PAO_2)
            a. Depressed alveolar ventilation

             (1) Central (neurologic disease, central nervous system [CNS] depressant medications)

             (2) Peripheral (neuromuscular disease, muscle relaxants)

        b. Increased respiratory dead space (drugs [atropine], hypotension, mechanical ventilation)

        c. Mechanical impairment of adequate ventilation (airway obstruction, thoracic cage disease)

        d. Diffusion hypoxemia

    3. Increased alveolar-arterial oxygen tension difference ($P[A - a]O_2$)

        a. Extrapulmonary

             (1) Right-to-left cardiac shunts (atrial or ventricular septal defects [ASD, VSD], tetralogy of Fallot)

             (2) Decreased mixed venous oxygenation saturation ($S\bar{v}O_2$)

        b. Intrapulmonary

             (1) V/Q mismatching (pulmonary edema, pulmonary embolism, contusion, aspiration, intrinsic lung disease)

             (2) Shunts (atelectasis, one-lung ventilation, endobronchial intubation, pneumothorax)

             (3) Impaired diffusion (intrinsic lung disease)

    4. Sampling error

  B. Anemic hypoxemia

    1. Low hemoglobin level

    2. High oxygen affinity hemoglobin (hemoglobin Yakima, hemoglobin Chesapeake)

    3. Shift of oxyhemoglobin dissociation curve (fetal hemoglobin, physiologic shift to the left)

  C. Toxic hypoxemia

    1. Carbon monoxide poisoning (carboxyhemoglobin)

    2. Methemoglobinemia

III. Toxic hypoxia—cyanide poisoning

DISCUSSION

As stated, oxygen transport is the product of cardiac output and oxygen content (multiplied by 10 for consistency of units):

$$O_2 \text{ transport} = \text{C.O.} \times CaO_2 \text{ (ml } O_2/\text{min)} \times 10$$

The oxygen transport index equals the oxygen transport divided by the body surface area, with a normal value of 550 to 650 ml/minute/m^2. CaO_2 is the number of milliliters of oxygen contained in 100 ml of blood. It can be calculated using the following equation:

$$CaO_2 = (1.37 \times Hb \times SaO_2) + (0.003 \times PaO_2)$$

where 1.37 = number of milliliters of oxygen bound to 1 g of fully saturated Hb

Hb = hemoglobin in grams/100 ml of blood

SaO_2 = percentage of oxyhemoglobin to total hemoglobin saturation

0.003 = solubility of oxygen in plasma (vol%/mm Hg)

PaO_2 = arterial partial pressure of oxygen in mm Hg

The normal CaO_2 is 18 to 20 vol%. Overall, tissue oxygenation is directly dependent on PaO_2, SaO_2, hemoglobin, and cardiac output; problems with any of these four parameters can lead to tissue hypoxia. A convenient way to divide these is shown in Table 1-1.

The initial step in evaluation is to obtain an arterial blood gas. Once laboratory error has been ruled out, a low PaO_2 indicates hypoxic hypoxemia, which accounts for the majority of cases of tissue hypoxia. The causes of hypoxic hypoxemia are numerous and generally include (1) low FiO_2, (2) reduced alveolar oxygen tension, and (3) increased alveolar-arterial oxygen tension difference.

A low FiO_2 in hypoxic hypoxemia may be caused by a cracked flowmeter or common manifold, line crossover, exhausted oxygen tanks, or failure to provide adequate oxygen flow

Table 1-1. Causes of Tissue Hypoxia: Classification Based on
Hemodynamic and Laboratory Parameters

	PaO_2	SaO_2	Hb	C.O.
Ischemic hypoxia	—	—	—	↓
Hypoxemic hypoxia				
Hypoxic hypoxemia	↓	↓	—	—
Anemic hypoxemia	—	—	↓	—
Toxic hypoxemia	—	↓	—	—
Toxic hypoxia	—	—	—	—

when nitrous oxide is used. A low FIO_2 can quickly be diagnosed by using an oxygen analyzer in the circuit.

The second cause of hypoxic hypoxemia is reduced alveolar oxygen tension (PAO_2). PAO_2 is the oxygen that exists at the blood-gas exchange surface in the lung and can be calculated using the alveolar oxygen equation:

$$PAO_2 = (PB - 47) FIO_2 - PaCO_2/0.8$$

where PB = barometric pressure
47 = water vapor pressure (mm Hg)

Therefore, any disorder that leads to an increased $PaCO_2$ will subsequently lead to a decreased PAO_2. These disorders include (1) alveolar hypoventilation due to drugs (sedatives, narcotics, muscle relaxants) or disease states (neuromuscular diseases, CNS disorders), (2) increased dead space (hypotension, atropine), and (3) mechanical impairment (airway obstruction). Atropine increases the intracellular concentration of cyclic guanosine monophosphate (CGMP) and therefore produces bronchodilation. Bronchodilation, by increasing physiologic dead space, can lead to relative alveolar hypoventilation. A rare cause of decreased PAO_2 is diffusion hypoxia, which can occur at the end of administration of a general anesthetic as nitrous oxide rapidly diffuses from the blood into the alveoli, thereby diluting the remaining oxygen. It is infrequently seen today, since 100% oxygen is routinely delivered at the end of a general anesthetic.

The third cause of hypoxic hypoxemia is increased alveolar-arterial oxygen tension difference [P(A − a)O_2]. P(A − a)O_2 is a measure of the efficiency of oxygen exchange. The greater this difference, the more impaired oxygen exchange is; it usually presents as a low PaO_2. This situation develops when there are abnormalities in the distribution of ventilation (V) to blood flow (Q). V/Q mismatching due to lung disease is the most common cause of low PaO_2; it may be exaggerated during general anesthesia due to impairment of hypoxic pulmonary vasoconstriction or alterations in respiratory mechanics. Disorders such as pulmonary edema, pulmonary embolus, or lung contusions may produce V/Q mismatching.

Three other causes of increased P(A − a)O_2 are shunts, decreased $S\bar{v}O_2$, and impaired oxygen diffusion. Shunts are one extreme of V/Q mismatching, when blood perfuses unventilated alveoli; it is characterized by the inability to increase PaO_2 when 100% oxygen is given. The most obvious examples of this process are right-to-left intracardiac shunts, as seen in ASD, VSD, and tetralogy of Fallot. Extrapulmonary shunts that occur in normal individuals include drainage from bronchial and thebesian veins. Intrapulmonary causes of shunts include one-lung ventilation using a double-lumen endotracheal tube, atelectasis, pneumothorax, and endobronchial intubation. Decreased $S\bar{v}O_2$ occurs when there is increased oxygen extraction at the tissue level, leading to a decreased oxygen reserve in the blood. Causes of increased extraction include decreased perfusion (reduced cardiac output) and increased oxygen consumption (fever, tissue repair). Impaired oxygen diffusion due to thickening of the alveolar-capillary basement membrane is a rare cause of low PaO_2. It is diagnosed by specialized pulmonary function tests using carbon monoxide diffusion.

The two other major divisions of hypoxemic hypoxia are anemic and toxic hypoxemia. Anemic hypoxemia occurs when the hemoglobin level is low or when its affinity for oxygen is increased. High affinity may be due to either abnormalities in the hemoglobin itself (hemoglobin Yakima) or shifts in the oxyhemoglobin dissociation curve, as in fetal hemoglobin or physiologic shift to the left secondary to alkalosis, low temperature, or low 2, 3-diphosphoglycerate.

Toxic hypoxemia occurs when there are alterations in hemoglobin's ability to unload oxygen (carbon monoxide poisoning, methemoglobinemia). Carbon monoxide has an affinity for hemoglobin 240 times greater than oxygen. The binding of carbon monoxide prevents the release of oxygen at the tissue level. Methemoglobinemia develops when the iron in the hemoglobin molecule is converted from the ferrous (Fe^{2+}) to the ferric (Fe^{3+}) form. This conversion increases the remaining hemoglobin affinity for oxygen, thus impairing the unloading of oxygen to tissues. Methemoglobinemia can be produced by drugs (sodium nitroprusside, prilocaine) in normal individuals or by phenacetin in patients with glucose-6-phosphate dehydrogenase (G-6-PD) deficiency.

The true oxygen content of arterial blood can be measured using a CO-Oximeter, which measures the total hemoglobin and the percentages of oxyhemoglobin, methemoglobin, and carboxyhemoglobin. In patients suspected of having carboxy- or methemoglobinemia, CO-oximetry is necessary, since the pulse oximeter may overestimate the saturation of hemoglobin with oxygen by reading the two abnormal forms as oxyhemoglobin.

The second major cause of inadequate tissue oxygenation is toxic hypoxia, primarily due to cyanide toxicity. In this disorder, cyanide binds to cytochrome oxidase in the mitochondria and inhibits electron transport, thereby causing cellular hypoxia. It may be suspected in patients receiving sodium nitroprusside who develop an unexplained metabolic acidosis. In these patients, the cardiac output, hemoglobin, PaO_2, CaO_2, and CO-oximetry may be normal.

The last major category is ischemic hypoxia due to inadequate blood flow and tissue perfusion. It may result from decreased cardiac output, as in congestive heart failure, or impaired blood flow to tissues, as with major arteriosclerotic vascular disease. In these cases, the oxygen content is usually normal. Diagnosis of decreased cardiac output may be aided by placing a pulmonary artery catheter and measuring cardiac output and $S\bar{v}O_2$.

It should be noted that one disease process may lead to tissue hypoxia by a number of the aforementioned mechanisms. An example is gram-negative septic shock. Patients with this condition may develop decreased cardiac output, increased oxygen consumption, peripheral and pulmonary shunts, and impaired pulmonary oxygen diffusion secondary to adult respiratory distress syndrome, all contributing in varying degrees to tissue hypoxia.

SELECTED READING

Foltz BD, Benumof JL: Mechanisms of hypoxemia and hypercapnia in the perioperative period. *Crit Care Clin* 3 : 269, 1987.

Laycock GJ, McNicol LR: Hypoxemia during induction of anaessia: An audit of children who underwent general anaesthesia for routine elective surgery. *Anaesthesia* 43 : 981, 1988.

2
Hypercapnia

DEFINITION

Hypercapnia is defined as an abnormal elevation in arterial carbon dioxide ($PaCO_2$) level, with normal values in adults ranging from 35 to 45 mm Hg. Since the lungs are the only route of carbon dioxide elimination, all hypercapnia is ultimately due to inadequate alveolar ventilation. However, the predisposing causes may be increased carbon dioxide production or decreased carbon dioxide elimination.

ETIOLOGY

I. Decreased elimination
   A. Inadequate minute ventilation (spontaneous or controlled)
   B. Depleted carbon dioxide absorber
   C. Rebreathing (stuck expiratory valve, inadequate flows with a semiopen circuit)
   D. Respiratory failure
   E. Chronic obstructive pulmonary disease (COPD)
   F. V/Q mismatching (pulmonary embolus, cardiac arrest)
II. Increased production
   A. Malignant hyperthermia
   B. Thyrotoxicosis
   C. Fever
   D. Total parenteral nutrition (TPN)
   E. Shivering
   F. Carbon dioxide insufflation (laparoscopic procedures)
   G. Sodium bicarbonate administration

DISCUSSION

First, the arterial pH must be evaluated to determine if the elevation in $PaCO_2$ is acute or chronic. A normal pH indicates a chronic condition (e.g., COPD), while a pH less than 7.35 suggests an acute process with concomitant respiratory acidosis. The end-tidal carbon dioxide ($ETCO_2$) can be used roughly to follow $PaCO_2$. However, discrepancies may arise due to ventilation-perfusion (V/Q) mismatching. In particular, if physiologic dead space (areas ventilated but not perfused) increases, the $ETCO_2$ will be much lower than the $PaCO_2$. This situation occurs with pulmonary embolism and cardiac arrest.

Overall, the most common cause for hypercapnia is decreased carbon dioxide elimination secondary to inadequate minute ventilation. It can occur in patients under general anesthesia who are spontaneously breathing, since halogenated anesthetics and narcotics blunt the respiratory center's responsiveness to carbon dioxide. Hypercapnia may also develop when patients are mechanically ventilated if the tidal volume or respiratory rates are too low. In either case, increasing the tidal volume or respiratory rate will return the $PaCO_2$ to normal levels. Rebreathing of expired gases due to an exhausted carbon dioxide absorber, stuck expiratory valve, or inadequate gas flow rates with semiopen circuits also will lead to an increase in $PaCO_2$. In these cases, a change in the color of the carbon dioxide absorber or the failure of the carbon dioxide waveform on the capnograph to return to baseline will help diagnose the problem (Fig. 2-1).

Overproduction of carbon dioxide is the second major predisposing cause of hypercapnia. Catabolic states, such as occur with fever, shivering, or TPN administration, are usually apparent during the initial preoperative evaluation. In severely ill patients, arterial blood gases should be drawn preoperatively to obtain baseline values of $PaCO_2$.

If the above causes of hypercapnia have been ruled out, the patient may have thyrotoxicosis or malignant hyperthermia.

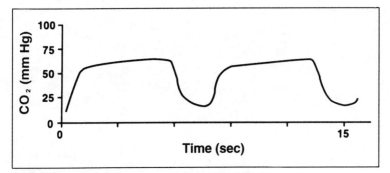

Figure 2-1. Capnogram showing rebreathing. The inspiratory valve was stuck, and during inspiration some of the expired gas was reinhaled. (From Gravenstein JS, Paulus DA: *Monitoring Ventilation and Gases*. In Gravenstein JS, Paulus DA [eds]: *Clinical Monitoring Practice*. Philadelphia: Lippincott, 1987.)

Although thyrotoxicosis can develop de novo, most cases arise in individuals with a history of hyperthyroidism or symptomatology compatible with it (recent weight loss, exophthalmos, enlarged thyroid). Of major concern is malignant hyperthermia, which cannot be ruled out by a negative personal or family history. If the index of suspicion is high, the patient should be treated with intravenous dantrolene and surgery stopped until further diagnostic studies can be done.

SELECTED READING

Foltz BD, Benumof JL: Mechanisms of hypoxemia and hypercapnia in the perioperative period. *Crit Care Clin* 3 : 269, 1987.
Weinberger SE, Schwartzstein RM, Weiss JM: Hypercapnia. *N Engl J Med* 321 : 1223, 1989.

3
Airway Obstruction

DEFINITION

Airway obstruction is defined as a blockage in the air passage that prevents gas movement; this blockage may be either partial or complete. Causes of airway obstruction can be divided into two major categories depending on whether the natural or an artificial airway is present.

ETIOLOGY

I. Natural airway
  A. Oropharynx
    1. Soft tissue obstruction (posterior tongue displacement)
    2. Foreign body (dentures, misplaced oral airway, vomitus)
    3. Pharyngeal abscess
    4. Pharyngeal packs
  B. Larynx
    1. Foreign body
    2. Laryngospasm
    3. Laryngeal edema
    4. Epiglottitis
    5. Tumor (papillomas, carcinoma)
    6. Bilateral damage to recurrent laryngeal nerves
    7. Laryngeal fracture
  C. Large airways
    1. Foreign body (tooth)
    2. Subglottic stenosis

3. Extrinsic compression (tumor [goiter], carotid hematoma)
4. Vomitus
5. Subglottic edema
6. Thick secretions
7. Clamping of major airway by surgeons

II. Endotracheal tube (ETT)/tracheostomy
   A. Kinked ETT
   B. Overinflation of cuff
   C. Foreign body
   D. ETT against carina or mucosa
   E. Endobronchial intubation
   F. Secretions or blood

DISCUSSION

As stated, airway obstruction can be partial or complete. Complete obstruction is usually obvious, as there is no air movement and breath sounds are absent. Actual air movement can be ascertained by placing a hand over the patient's mouth or observing fogging of the face mask; if an ETT is present, there should be movement of the reservoir bag or spirometer. Retraction of the intercostal muscles or tugging of the diaphragm should not be interpreted as adequate ventilation. Partial obstruction is usually indicated by a variety of noisy airway sounds (crowing, stridor, wheezing). Gas exchange may be of sufficient amounts to prevent a decrease in oxygen saturation. Signs of airway obstruction are listed in Table 3-1.

In patients with airway obstruction, diagnosis and treatment often occur simultaneously. The most frequent cause of obstruction during the induction or emergence phase of anesthesia is posterior displacement of the tongue due to soft tissue relaxation. Partial obstruction is characterized by snoring; treatment consists of anterior displacement of the mandible (placing fingers behind angle of mandible and pulling forward)

Table 3-1. Signs of Airway Obstruction

Spontaneous ventilation
  Increasing ventilatory effort (reflex due to hypercarbia, hypoxia)
  Retraction of intercostal, supraclavicular, and abdominal tissues
  Reduced or absent breath sounds over lung fields
  Abnormal breath sounds due to turbulence, especially in upper
    airway
  Reduced or absent exchange of gas (i.e., absence of sound,
    temperature change, moisture condensation at lips or in
    endotracheal tube; reduced or absent movement of reservoir
    bag; spirometer records low or no tidal volume)
  Signs of hypoxemia and hypercarbia
Positive-pressure ventilation
  High lung inflation pressure
  Reservoir bag does not empty (i.e., inspiratory obstruction) or
    does not refill normally (i.e., expiratory obstruction)
  Absence of condensation in endotracheal tube
  Reduced or absent breath sounds over lung fields and in
    breathing circuit
  Little or no movement of thorax or abdominal wall with
    application and release of positive pressure
  Signs of hypoxemia and hypercarbia

Source: From Hug CC Jr.: Monitoring. In Miller RD (ed): *Anesthesia*, 2nd
ed. New York: Churchill Livingstone, 1986.

and slight extension of the neck. If unsuccessful, placement of an oral or nasal airway is usually effective in relieving the obstruction. However, the obstruction may worsen if the oral airway is placed without proper positioning of the tongue. Other causes of oropharyngeal obstruction include foreign bodies such as dentures or vomitus. A pharyngeal pack may have been placed during upper airway surgery, such as a tonsillectomy; failure to remove it may lead to obstruction. The presence of a pharyngeal or peritonsillar abscess is usually known preoperatively.

At the level of the larynx, the most common cause of obstruction is laryngospasm. This reflex closure of the vocal cords is almost always due either to manipulation of the airway in the absence of adequate anesthesia or to irritation of the larynx by secretions or blood. The first indication of laryngospasm is a high-pitched, "crowing" sound. Treatment consists of suctioning the airway, thrusting the jaw forward, applying positive pressure to the airway, and if necessary, administering a rapid-acting muscle relaxant. Other causes of laryngeal obstruction include (1) foreign bodies, (2) laryngeal edema secondary to surgery, trauma, or rarely, hereditary angioneurotic edema, and (3) a tumor in the airway. An airway tumor may cause obstruction after induction, since general anesthesia can cause relaxation of the soft tissues and therefore collapse of supporting structures.

Two rare causes of airway obstruction are bilateral damage to the recurrent laryngeal nerves and laryngeal fractures. Nerve damage may occur during a thyroidectomy and present postoperatively as severe obstruction; this obstruction worsens when respiration is active, as occurs when patients are anxious. Laryngeal fractures are usually secondary to motor vehicle accidents in which the driver's neck hits the top of the steering wheel. Patients can have a variety of outcomes, depending on the level of the fracture; they may die instantly, present with airway obstruction, or develop subcutaneous emphysema and stridor.

Obstruction below the level of the vocal cords may be secondary to a number of causes. Foreign bodies, such as peanuts, hot dogs, or coins, are common causes in children between 6 and 36 months old. In most cases, the object is radiolucent and the only symptoms may be recurrent lower respiratory tract infections or localized wheezing on physical examination. If an intubation was difficult, a dislodged tooth may become embedded in a large bronchus. Vomitus or thick secretions may become impacted in a major bronchus and require suctioning or bronchoscopy to remove. Extrinsic compression due to a tumor or hematoma is usually apparent. Immediately following extubation, subglottic edema may cause narrowing of the tracheal diameter, a condition that becomes more significant in infants and children who have smaller tracheas. If intubation was prolonged or if a tracheostomy was placed, the patient may develop subglottic stenosis.

If an endotracheal tube or tracheostomy is present, first a suction catheter should be passed to remove any secretions or blood and to determine if the tube is kinked. Second, the tracheal cuff should be deflated and reinflated just until a seal is obtained. Third, an endobronchial intubation should be ruled out by assuring bilateral breath sounds; if uncertain, a chest radiograph should be ordered. Last, if these measures are not diagnostic, a bronchoscope should be passed through the tube to look for causes of obstruction, such as foreign bodies.

SELECTED READING

Pincus RL: Nasopharyngeal obstruction. *Otolaryngol Clin North Am* 22 : 367, 1989.

Zalzal GH: Stridor and airway compromise. *Pediatr Clin North Am* 36 : 1389, 1989.

4
Difficult Intubation

DEFINITION

Endotracheal intubation is performed routinely after induction of general anesthesia. Although easily accomplished in the majority of cases, in some patients intubation is difficult, if not impossible. Occasionally, intubation is difficult because of poor clinical technique on the part of the laryngoscopist or malfunctioning equipment. In most instances, however, the problem lies with the patient's anatomy or underlying disease process.

ETIOLOGY
I. Patient's anatomy
   A. Small mouth opening
   B. Micrognathia
   C. Maxillary overbite
   D. High vaulted palate
   E. Obesity
   F. Short, muscular neck
   G. Anterior larynx
   H. Limited mobility (neck, temporomandibular joint [TMJ])
   I. Large tongue
II. Disease process
   A. Scars (burns, radiation, previous surgery)
   B. Maxillofacial trauma
   C. Prior tracheostomy
   D. Cervical spine injury/instability
   E. Abscesses (peritonsillar, Ludwig's angina)

F. Hematoma
G. Epiglottitis
H. Rheumatoid arthritis
I. Ankylosing spondylitis
J. Tumors (laryngeal, pharyngeal, enlarged thyroid)
K. Bleeding (post-tonsillectomy)
L. Laryngeal edema/injury
M. Diabetic "stiff joint" syndrome
N. Pregnancy

DISCUSSION

Clinical evaluation of the patient's airway prior to induction
of general anesthesia is one of the most important aspects of
the physical examination performed by the anesthesiologist.
Initially, the patient should be questioned about known problems with intubation, and records from previous anesthetics
should be reviewed. Next, the patient's mouth and pharynx
should be examined for (1) limited opening, (2) micrognathia,
(3) maxillary overbite, and (4) high arched palate. Inability
to easily visualize the tonsillar pillars, uvula, and soft palate
increases the likelihood of a difficult intubation. Fiberoptic
laryngoscopy may be helpful in further evaluation of the airway, particularly when tumors are present. However, ability
to visualize the vocal cords with a fiberoptic laryngoscope
does not imply intubation will be without difficulty, since
induction of anesthesia will cause muscle relaxation and collapse of supporting structures. The mobility of the patient's
neck and TMJ should be evaluated; both obese and short,
muscular necks may have limited mobility.

Underlying disease processes may contribute to or directly
cause a difficult intubation. These processes include (1) limited mouth opening (scars, TMJ dysfunction), (2) cervical
spine pathology (subluxation, ankylosing spondylitis, diabetic "stiff joint" syndrome), (3) infections (epiglottitis, peritonsillar abscesses), (4) maxillofacial or laryngeal trauma or

tumors, (6) bleeding (e.g., post-tonsillectomy), and (7) hematomas. Mandibular fractures may limit jaw mobility either due to pain and trismus or anatomic derangements of the TMJ. Rheumatoid arthritis can involve the TMJ, cervical spine, or arytenoid cartilages, predisposing to difficulties with laryngoscopy and intubation. Patients with juvenile-onset diabetes of greater than 10 years' duration may have limited mobility of their atlanto-occipital joint, making orotracheal intubation impossible. Lastly, some women may be more difficult to intubate when pregnant because of either upper airway edema or large pendulous breasts.

If a difficult intubation is anticipated, certain steps should be taken to make the situation safer for the patient and easier for the laryngoscopist. A variety of laryngoscope blades should be available, as should other skilled personnel. The patient should be preoxygenated with 100% oxygen prior to any attempts at intubation. Sedation and topical anesthesia to the tongue may allow for brief laryngoscopy prior to induction to see if any portions of the larynx can be visualized. Other alternatives include blind nasal or fiberoptic intubation and intubation over a retrograde wire passed through the cricothyroid membrane. If these measures are unsuccessful, and if mask ventilation cannot be done, cricothyroidotomy or percutaneous transtracheal jet ventilation may be necessary to ensure adequate oxygenation and ventilation until a more secure airway can be established.

SELECTED READING

Benumof JL: Management of the difficult or impossible airway. *41st Annual Refresher Course Lectures and Clinical Update Program* American Society of Anesthesiologists. Lecture 163, pp 1–7.

Cote C: How to manage the difficult pediatric airway. *41st Annual Refresher Course Lectures and Clinical Update Program.* Lecture 262, American Society of Anesthesiologists, pp 1–7.

Shorten GD, Roberts JT: The prediction of a difficult intubation. *Anesthesiol Clin North Am* 9 : 63, 1991.

5
Increased Peak Inspiratory Pressure

DEFINITION

Peak inspiratory pressure (PIP) is that pressure generated by a set tidal volume at maximum inspiration. The baseline PIP may be elevated due to obesity or restrictive lung disease. Concern arises when the baseline level is normal and then increases intraoperatively. Increases in PIP may be due to problems with the endotracheal tube (ETT) or tracheostomy, lungs, or chest wall.

ETIOLOGY
   I. Endotracheal tube/tracheostomy
      A. Kinked or occluded ETT or tracheostomy (cuff over-inflated, nitrous oxide expanding cuff)
      B. Endobronchial intubation
      C. ETT against carina
      D. Light anesthesia (patient breathing against ETT)
  II. Lungs
      A. Tension pneumothorax
      B. Bronchospasm
      C. Overinflation of lungs (tidal volume too large)
      D. Pulmonary edema
      E. Adult respiratory distress syndrome (ARDS)
      F. Trendelenburg's position (abdominal contents compressing lungs)
 III. Chest wall
      A. Chest wall rigidity secondary to narcotics
      B. Surgeon leaning on chest wall
      C. Instruments placed on chest

DISCUSSION

Several steps should be taken to diagnose the cause of increased PIP. First, the endotracheal tube should be examined for kinks and a suction catheter passed to rule out occlusion (e.g., overinflated cuff overlying the tip) or to remove secretions. If the endotracheal tube cuff is inflated with air, the volume may increase two- to threefold if surrounded by a high concentration of nitrous oxide. Also, the depth of the ETT placement should be checked to ensure the tip is not against the carina or in the right mainstem bronchus. Second, one needs to be certain that no individual or heavy instruments are leaning on the chest wall. Next, auscultation of the chest may reveal wheezing (bronchospasm), rales (pulmonary edema, ARDS), or unilateral breath sounds (tension pneumothorax, endobronchial intubation).

If the above are negative, the cause of increased PIP may be insufficient anesthesia. High-dose narcotic techniques using fentanyl or sufentanil can cause chest wall rigidity in the absence of adequate muscle relaxation. A patient who is lightly anesthetized may breathe or cough against the endotracheal tube, leading to an abrupt increase of the PIP. Either situation can be corrected by deepening the level of anesthesia or administering a neuromuscular blocking agent.

SELECTED READING

Katz J: Management of intra-operative ventilatory emergencies. *39th Annual Refresher Course Lectures and Clinical Update Program.* American Society of Anesthesiologists. Lecture 265, pp 1–7.

Marini JJ: Monitoring during mechanical ventilation. *Clin Chest Med* 9 : 73, 1988.

6
Hypocapnia

DEFINITION

Hypocapnia, defined as an arterial $PaCO_2$ less than 35 mm Hg, is secondary to alveolar hyperventilation. The causes of alveolar hyperventilation and hypocapnia may be divided into acute or chronic, based on the arterial pH and serum bicarbonate level (HCO_3^-).

ETIOLOGY

I. Acute (elevated pH, decreased HCO_3^-)
  A. Mechanical hyperventilation, acute
  B. Acute hyperventilation syndrome (anxiety)
  C. Central nervous system injury or disease (tumor, encephalitis)
  D. Arterial hypoxemia, acute (pneumonia, asthma)
  E. Gram-negative sepsis
  F. Hyperthermia
  G. Salicylate overdose
  H. Exercise

II. Chronic (normal pH, decreased HCO_3^-)
  A. Arterial hypoxemia, chronic (pulmonary fibrosis, cyanotic heart disease)
  B. Pregnancy
  C. Hepatic cirrhosis
  D. Pulmonary vascular disease
  E. Mechanical hyperventilation, chronic

DISCUSSION

Acute or chronic hypocapnia can be distinguished by obtaining an arterial pH and bicarbonate level. Acute hypocapnia produces an elevated pH due to partial compensation by plasma bicarbonate; the bicarbonate level falls only about 2 mmol/liter for each 10 mm Hg reduction in $PaCO_2$. With chronic hypocapnia, compensation is much more complete, as the decreased $PaCO_2$ inhibits renal tubular resorption of and generation of bicarbonate. In this case, the pH is near normal, while the bicarbonate level is reduced 4 to 5 mmol/ liter for each 10 mm Hg decrease in $PaCO_2$.

Acute hypocapnia and associated respiratory alkalosis may be detrimental to the patient. Alkalosis causes a decrease in serum ionized calcium and directly enhances neuromuscular excitability, which may trigger tetany. Severe respiratory alkalosis may cause cerebral vasospasm, which can lead to confusion and loss of consciousness. Treatment of hypocapnia is directed at eliminating the underlying cause.

The patient's history and physical examination may indicate the causes of hypocapnia. These include fever, pregnancy, asthmatic attack, central nervous system disease, and salicylate overdose. Acute hyperventilation syndrome is characterized by perioral numbness and light-headedness. Laboratory studies may reveal arterial hypoxemia, hepatic failure, or sepsis, all of which may lead to hyperventilation.

Excessive mechanical ventilation is seen in both the operating room and intensive care unit and is a common cause of hypocapnia. If allowed to persist for 24 hours or more, the pH will normalize as the serum bicarbonate falls, a condition seen in patients being hyperventilated to help control elevated intracranial pressure.

SELECTED READING

Nunn JF: Carbon dioxide. In *Applied Respiratory Physiology*, 3rd ed. London: Butterworth, 1987. Pp 207–234.

7
Intraoperative Wheezing

DEFINITION

Wheezing is defined as a high-pitched whistling sound made during breathing. It may be secondary to airway obstruction or bronchospasm. Bronchospasm is the spasmodic contraction of smooth muscles in the bronchial wall. It should be noted that asthma is a distinct subset of bronchospasm (i.e., "not all wheezing is asthma"); it is due to an intrinsic increase in airway responsiveness to a variety of stimuli. As only a small percentage of cases of intraoperative wheezing is due to asthma, the etiology needs to be elucidated so appropriate interventions can be instituted. The etiology of intraoperative wheezing falls into two general categories: (1) extrinsic or primary nonpulmonary disorders or (2) intrinsic or primary pulmonary disorders.

ETIOLOGY
I. Extrinsic (primary nonpulmonary disorders)
   A. "Light" anesthesia
   B. Endobronchial intubation
   C. Endotracheal tube against carina
   D. Pneumothorax
   E. Mechanical obstruction of endotracheal tube (kinking, secretions, overinflation of cuff)
   F. Inhaling foreign body or substance (baralyme)
   G. Histamine release secondary to drugs (d-tubocurarine, morphine, sodium pentothal)
   H. Pulmonary edema
   I. Pulmonary embolus

     J. Allergic reaction

     K. Carcinoid syndrome

     L. Aspiration of gastric contents

     M. Predominance of parasympathetic tone (following anticholinergic drugs or nonselective beta-blockers)

II. Intrinsic (primary pulmonary disorders)

     A. IgE-mediated asthma

     B. Aspirin-induced asthma (benzoic acid from local anesthetics)

     C. Exercise-induced asthma (ventilating with cool, dry air)

     D. Chronic obstructive pulmonary disease (COPD)

DISCUSSION

Initial differentiation begins with the patient's past medical history. IgE-mediated, aspirin- or exercise-induced asthma may be the cause of the wheezing. A patient with a long history of cigarette smoking may have asthmatic bronchitis. Other conditions to consider are a history of congestive heart failure or fluid overload (pulmonary edema), prolonged bed rest (pulmonary embolus), and carcinoid tumor (carcinoid syndrome).

In the majority of patients who do not have a history of underlying lung disease, the etiology of wheezing is more likely extrinsic causes. In these cases, it is essential to determine the time course. Wheezing occurring at the induction of general anesthesia could be secondary to (1) aspiration of gastric contents, (2) "light" anesthesia with placement of a foreign body in the airway (i.e., endotracheal tube) and reflex bronchoconstriction, (3) endobronchial intubation, or (4) mechanical obstruction of the endotracheal tube. Wheezing that begins shortly after administration of a drug could be due to direct histamine release, as occurs with d-tubocurarine or morphine, or an allergic reaction secondary to an antibiotic. If wheezing develops following chest trauma or central venous access placement, a pneumothorax must be ruled out.

Interventions will depend on the most likely etiology. Initially, one must ensure adequate oxygenation; supplemental oxygen should be administered to all patients and either arterial blood gases or pulse oximetry should be monitored. The next step is to rule out mechanical obstruction of the endotracheal tube by passing a suction catheter down it. The tracheal cuff should be deflated and reinflated until the air leak has just disappeared. Physical examination should reveal unequal breath sounds (endobronchial intubation, pneumothorax), deviated trachea (pneumothorax), or rales (pulmonary edema). A portable chest radiograph should be obtained if the diagnosis is unclear and the patient is relatively stable. Pulmonary embolism requires more specific testing for diagnosis than is available in the operating room.

The most common cause of bronchospasm is inadequate depth of anesthesia for the particular stimulus. The situation occurs in both normal patients and patients with asthma. Optimizing the level of anesthesia with volatile agents may reduce or resolve the bronchospasm by depression of parasympathetic-mediated bronchoconstrictive reflexes or by direct relaxation of smooth muscle. Intravenous ketamine may be effective, either by deepening the level of anesthesia or by bronchodilating actions related to its sympathomimetic properties. Additional muscle relaxants may be needed if the patient is breathing or coughing against the endotracheal tube. If bronchospasm persists, drugs directed at the airways themselves will be needed. These drugs include (1) beta-adrenergic agonist agents, such as albuterol, administered directly into the inspiratory limb of the anesthesia circuit (these drugs may not work if bronchospasm severely impairs ventilation), (2) epinephrine, subcutaneously or intravenously, (3) aminophylline, given by continuous intravenous infusion, and (4) intravenous corticosteroids. Other treatment modalities include (1) humidification of gases in patients with exercise-induced asthma, (2) removal of foreign substances, and (3) furosemide and possibly inotropic drugs for pulmonary edema.

SELECTED READING

Bishop M: Bronchospasm: Managing and avoiding a potential anesthetic disaster. *41st Annual Refresher Course Lectures and Clinical Update Program.* American Society of Anesthesiologists. Lecture 272, pp 1–6.

Kingston HG, Hirshman CA: Perioperative management of the patient with asthma. *Anesth Analg* 63 : 844, 1984.

8
End-Tidal Nitrogen

DEFINITION

The development of mass spectrometry has allowed the monitoring of end-tidal gas concentrations. The detection of end-tidal nitrogen (ETN_2) indicates the presence of room air in the circuit. Nitrogen entry may occur at any point from the anesthesia machine to the patient.

ETIOLOGY

1. Inadequate preoxygenation/denitrogenation
2. Leak in anesthesia machine (cracked flowmeter, poor seal around carbon dioxide cannister)
3. Leak around endotracheal tube cuff
4. Use of air from air flowmeter
5. Nitrogen dissolved in body fluids
6. Venous air embolism

DISCUSSION

End-tidal nitrogen detected immediately after intubation is due to inadequate preoxygenation during induction. A small amount of end-tidal nitrogen may be present for several minutes after intubation, since up to a liter of nitrogen gas is dissolved in body fluids and slowly dissipates into the blood and alveoli.

Leaks in the anesthesia circuit can occur at multiple points. Many can be discovered by performing a high-pressure check;

the most common site is around the carbon dioxide cannister. Leaks can develop in the machine itself (e.g., secondary to a cracked flowmeter); these problems are more difficult to detect and may require special servicing by trained personnel. If the high-pressure check is normal, the nitrogen could be entering around a cuffed endotracheal tube with an inadequate seal; this problem is corrected by adding air to the cuff.

The most important situation to rule out is venous air embolism (VAE). VAE may occur in any surgical procedure but is most frequently encountered in sitting craniotomies and pelvic surgeries (including cesarean sections). A high index of suspicion, along with a decreased end-tidal carbon dioxide, hypotension, and cardiac arrhythmias, will help to diagnose VAE. Treatment includes (1) administering 100% oxygen, (2) preventing further entrainment of room air, (3) placing the patient in the left lateral decubitus position (when possible) to help remove the air block, and (4) supporting the cardiovascular system.

SELECTED READING

Eisenkraft J: What anesthesiologists should know about mass spectrometry and intraoperative gas monitoring. *ASA Regional Refresher Course, Washington DC*. American Society of Anesthesiologists. Lecture 109, 1989. Pp 1–8.

Matjasko MJ, Gunselman J, Delaney J, Mackenzie CI: Sources of nitrogen in the anesthesia circuit. *Anesthesiology* 65 : 229, 1986.

9
Cyanosis

DEFINITION

Cyanosis is a bluish discoloration of the skin, lips, or mucous membranes, resulting from an excessive concentration of reduced hemoglobin or hemoglobin derivatives in the blood. It may be classified as central or peripheral. Central cyanosis is produced as a result of either arterial desaturation or abnormal hemoglobin. Peripheral cyanosis develops when excessive amounts of reduced hemoglobin collect in venous blood; the underlying causes are peripheral vasoconstriction and reduced blood flow, which lead to extensive oxygen extraction at the capillary level. Generally, cyanosis becomes apparent when the absolute amount of reduced hemoglobin is greater than 5 g/dl. However, when cyanosis is due to nonfunctional hemoglobin, smaller quantities are needed; as little as 1.5 g/dl of methemoglobin or 0.5 g/dl of sulfhemoglobin may produce cyanosis.

ETIOLOGY

I. Central cyanosis
  A. Decreased arterial oxygen saturation
    1. Low oxygen concentration in inspired air (FiO_2)/ diffusion hypoxemia
    2. Shunts
      a. Congenital heart disease (tetralogy of Fallot, transposition of great vessels, Ebstein's anomaly)
      b. Intrapulmonary shunts (cirrhosis)

3. Pulmonary disease
   a. Acute (pulmonary embolism, pneumonia, pneumothorax)
   b. Chronic obstructive or restrictive lung diseases
   B. Hemoglobin abnormalities
   1. Methemoglobinemia
   2. Sulfhemoglobinemia
   3. Low oxygen affinity hemoglobin variants (hemoglobin Kansas)
II. Peripheral cyanosis
   A. Reduced cardiac output (congestive heart failure)
   B. Shock
   C. Cold exposure (generalized, Raynaud's phenomenon)
   D. Arterial occlusion
   E. Venous occlusion

DISCUSSION

The history and physical examination are important when approaching a patient with cyanosis. Cyanosis present since birth is usually due to congenital heart disease; rarely, congenital methemoglobinemia is the cause. A history of smoking, dyspnea, wheezing, or sputum production is commonly seen with pulmonary disease. Drugs or chemicals that may produce methemoglobinemia or sulfhemoglobinemia include phenacetin, nitrates, nitrites, quinones, sulfonamides, and aniline dyes. Patients with hepatic cirrhosis often develop intrapulmonary shunts, which lead to arterial hypoxemia and cyanosis. Other historical findings that should be elicited include claudication (arterial occlusion), thrombophlebitis (venous obstruction), and pallor followed by redness after fingers are exposed to cold (Raynaud's phenomenon). A patient recovering from general anesthesia may be receiving a hypoxic gas mixture or may have diffusion hypoxemia as the cause.

Certain findings on physical examination will help distinguish central from peripheral cyanosis. With central cyanosis, the skin and mucous membranes are discolored, while only the distal extremities or nail beds are involved in peripheral cyanosis. Clubbing is common in severe central cyanosis due to cardiac or pulmonary disease. Murmurs are usually present with congenital heart lesions. Auscultation of the lungs may reveal unequal breath sounds (pneumothorax), rales (pulmonary edema), or areas of consolidation (pneumonia). Lastly, warming a cyanotic extremity may increase peripheral blood flow and help abolish peripheral cyanosis due to cold exposure.

Laboratory studies that may provide diagnostic information include (1) complete blood count (erythrocytosis may develop in patients with congenital heart disease or chronic lung disorders), (2) arterial blood gases (the PaO_2 is low in all cases of central cyanosis, while it is usually normal in peripheral cyanosis), and (3) chest radiograph (for evidence of chronic lung disease or congestive heart failure). If a hemoglobin abnormality is suspected, electrophoresis of a hemoglobin sample should be obtained. An extremely rare hemoglobin mutant, hemoglobin Kansas, causes central cyanosis due to a low hemoglobin affinity for oxygen.

SELECTED READING

Martin L, Khalil H: How much reduced hemoglobin is necessary to generate central cyanosis? *Chest* 9 : 182, 1990.
Timmins AC, Morgan GA: Argyria or cyanosis? *Anaesthesia* 43 : 755, 1988.

10
Hemoptysis

DEFINITION

Hemoptysis is defined as the expectoration of blood or blood-streaked sputum. Although its presence indicates underlying pathology, from 5 to 15 percent of the cases of gross hemoptysis remain undiagnosed despite extensive evaluation. A variety of pulmonary, cardiovascular, and miscellaneous disorders can produce hemoptysis.

ETIOLOGY

  I. Pulmonary
   A. Infectious (chronic bronchitis, bronchiectasis, tuberculosis, lung abscess, pneumonia)
   B. Neoplastic (carcinoma, bronchial adenoma)
   C. Traumatic (lung contusion, foreign body)
   D. Pulmonary embolism with infarction
   E. Autoimmune (Goodpasture's syndrome)
 II. Cardiovascular
   A. Left ventricular failure with pulmonary edema
   B. Pulmonary hypertension (primary, recurrent pulmonary emboli, mitral stenosis)
   C. Pulmonary artery rupture
   D. Arteriovenous malformations
III. Miscellaneous
   A. Hemorrhagic diathesis
   B. Upper airway trauma (difficult intubation, post-tonsillectomy)
   C. Upper gastrointestinal bleeding
   D. Wegener's granulomatosis

DISCUSSION

The initial step in diagnosis is to determine that the blood is originating from the lower respiratory tract and not from the gastrointestinal tract or nasopharynx. Upper gastrointestinal bleeding may be mistaken for hemoptysis if the patient aspirated blood. Upper respiratory tract bleeding may stem from direct trauma (nasogastric tube insertion, difficult intubation), upper airway surgery (posttonsillectomy), or inflammatory disorders (Wegener's granulomatosis). A patient with a bleeding diathesis (e.g., coagulation factor or platelet defects) may be prone to bleeding following upper airway manipulations.

True hemoptysis results from disorders in the pulmonary or cardiovascular systems. The history is critical and often suggests specific diagnoses. The most likely causes are pulmonary infections and include bronchiectasis (particularly in children with cystic fibrosis), chronic bronchitis, and tuberculosis. Neoplasia is the second most common reason. Lung cancer heads the list in patients with a history of heavy tobacco abuse and weight loss; it accounts for 20 percent of all cases of hemoptysis. Recurrent hemoptysis in a young, otherwise healthy female favors the diagnosis of bronchial adenoma. Pulmonary embolism with infarction can occur in patients with certain risk factors, such as solid tumors, prolonged bed rest, or oral contraceptive use. Autoimmune diseases can directly affect the pulmonary parenchyma and produce bleeding; Goodpasture's syndrome is the most common and is associated with involvement of the renal glomerulus.

Of the cardiovascular disorders, left ventricular failure with pulmonary edema is the most common cause; it is characterized by abundant quantities of pink, frothy sputum. A variety of disease states can lead to pulmonary hypertension, including mitral stenosis and recurrent pulmonary embolism. Primary pulmonary hypertension can develop in young, previously healthy females and is a diagnosis of exclusion.

Arteriovenous malformations occur in patients with Osler-Weber-Rendu disease and can produce massive hemoptysis when ruptured.

Other causes of hemoptysis include trauma, either secondary to lung contusion or foreign body in the airway, and pulmonary artery rupture. Pulmonary artery rupture, a rare phenomenon, can occur in patients with a pulmonary artery catheter. The risk is greatly increased if the catheter tip is advanced too far, if the balloon is overinflated, or if the patient has pulmonary artery hypertension. Diagnosis is usually obvious, as the patient develops massive hemoptysis after inflation of the catheter balloon; it is often fatal.

Physical examination may give clues to the diagnosis. Findings of importance include pleural friction rub (pulmonary embolism with infarction), clubbing (bronchogenic carcinoma), localized wheezing (foreign body), and diastolic rumble (mitral stenosis). As previously stated, the upper airway should be thoroughly examined for evidence of bleeding.

After the history and physical examination, certain diagnostic studies should be performed. The most important is a chest radiograph, particularly if the etiology is suspected to be neoplastic or infectious. Findings include tumors, infiltrates with pneumonia, or air fluid levels with lung abscesses. If nondiagnostic, the next step is evaluation of the airway with fiberoptic bronchoscopy. This procedure is most beneficial when the bleeding is scant, as occurs with chronic bronchitis. Other studies that may need to be performed include echocardiogram for mitral stenosis, cytology for occult malignancy, ventilation-perfusion scans for pulmonary embolism, pulmonary angiography for recurrent pulmonary embolism or arteriovenous malformations, and coagulation profiles for bleeding diathesis. Bronchography is indicated to rule out bronchiectasis in patients with recurrent bleeding or recurrent infections whose chest radiograph is normal. Open lung biopsy may be required if the diagnosis is unclear or if Goodpasture's syndrome or an occult infectious process is suspected.

SELECTED READING

Haponik EF, Chin R: Hemoptysis: Clinicians' perspectives. *Chest* 97 : 469, 1990.

Wedzicha JA, Pearson MC: Management of massive hemoptysis. *Respir Med* 84 : 9, 1990.

11
Dyspnea

DEFINITION

Dyspnea is defined as an abnormally uncomfortable awareness of breathing with the subjective complaint of shortness
of breath. It is due to excessive work of breathing; either the
lungs and chest wall are less compliant or the resistance to air
flow is increased. The etiology of dyspnea can be divided into
pulmonary or nonpulmonary causes.

ETIOLOGY
I. Pulmonary
   A. Airway obstruction (tumor, laryngeal edema, foreign
      body)
   B. Bronchospasm
   C. Restrictive lung disease (sarcoidosis, rheumatoid
      lung, pneumoconioses, alveolar proteinosis)
   D. Emphysema
   E. Pulmonary embolism (acute, recurrent)
   F. Bronchitis (chronic, acute)
   G. Pneumonia
   H. Pneumothorax
   I. Pulmonary edema (cardiogenic [congestive heart
      failure], noncardiogenic)
II. Nonpulmonary
   A. Chest wall
      1. Kyphoscoliosis
      2. Pectus excavatum
      3. Obesity
      4. Pain (thoracotomy, subcostal incisions)

B. Respiratory muscles
   1. Neuromuscular disease (myasthenia gravis, amyotrophic lateral sclerosis, poliomyelitis, Guillain-Barré syndrome)
   2. Residual muscle relaxants
   3. Regional anesthesia (subarachnoid, epidural blockade)
C. Poor physical conditioning
D. Hyperventilation

DISCUSSION

In diagnosing the cause of dyspnea, the first step is to determine whether the onset is acute or chronic. Chronic dyspnea is present preoperatively, and the cause can usually be discovered by history and physical examination. Most often, it is due to (1) chronic obstructive or restrictive lung disease, such as emphysema or pneumoconioses, (2) chest wall deformities, such as kyphoscoliosis or pectus excavatum, (3) obesity, or (4) poor physical conditioning. Physical examination may reveal a thin patient with distant breath sounds and an enlarged chest with emphysema, wheezing with chronic asthma, or cyanosis with chronic bronchitis. Rare causes of dyspnea include anemia and hyperthyroidism; hyperventilation syndrome as a cause of dyspnea is a diagnosis of exclusion.

Causes of acute dyspnea can be superimposed on chronic dyspnea or may develop independently. Recent fever and increased cough and sputum production indicate pneumonia or acute bronchitis; in addition, infection commonly exacerbates asthma and congestive heart failure. Foreign body aspiration may occur in children or in patients with impaired level of consciousness, such as alcoholics or drug abusers. Wheezing may be due to underlying bronchospastic disease or a number of other causes (see Chap. 7). Airway obstruction

may be secondary to tumor or laryngeal edema. Pneumothorax may (1) develop spontaneously in tall, thin individuals, (2) follow central line placement, or (3) present after
recent chest trauma. Acute pulmonary embolism (PE) should
be suspected in patients immobilized, on prolonged bed rest,
after surgery, or taking oral contraceptives. Recurrent PE
may produce pulmonary vascular occlusive disease with pulmonary hypertension and chronic dyspnea.

Pulmonary edema, either cardiogenic or noncardiogenic,
may produce acute dyspnea. If cardiogenic in origin, symptoms include orthopnea (dyspnea while lying flat) and paroxysmal nocturnal dyspnea (PND). PND, also known as cardiac
asthma, is characterized by severe attacks of shortness of
breath that awaken the patient from sleep. Patients with
either orthopnea or PND give a history of improvement of
dyspnea with sitting upright.

Laboratory studies that may be beneficial in diagnosis
include chest radiograph (pneumonia, congestive heart failure), arterial blood gases, electrocardiogram (myocardial
infarction with pulmonary edema), and complete blood
count (anemia, leukocytosis). Pulmonary function tests are
helpful to discover causes of chronic dyspnea. Ventilation-
perfusion scanning or pulmonary angiography may be
needed to diagnose acute or recurrent PE.

Several causes of acute dyspnea occur specifically in the
perioperative period. They are related to the location of the
surgical incision or the anesthetic itself. Thoracic or sub-
costal incisions often produce so much pain that the patient
is unable to take a deep breath; this resolves with adequate
analgesia. The possibility of residual muscle relaxation
should be immediately evaluated and, if necessary, additional anticholinesterase drugs given. High epidural or subarachnoid anesthesia may produce a sensation of shortness
of breath due to lack of sensory feedback from the lungs;
this complaint often resolves with reassurance.

SELECTED READING

Cockcroft A, Adams L, Guz A: Assessment of breathlessness. *Q J Med* 72 : 669, 1989.

Sweer L, Zwillich CW: Dyspnea in the patient with chronic obstructive pulmonary disease: Etiology and management. *Clin Chest Med* 11 : 417, 1990.

12
Pulmonary Edema

DEFINITION

Pulmonary edema is defined as the abnormal extravascular accumulation of fluid in the pulmonary interstitium and alveoli. It is primarily due to either increased pulmonary capillary pressure (cardiogenic pulmonary edema) or increased pulmonary capillary permeability (noncardiogenic pulmonary edema). In addition, four other forms have not been directly related to either mechanism, and their precise pathophysiology remains unclear.

ETIOLOGY

   I. Increased pulmonary capillary pressure (cardiogenic)
      A. Left ventricular dysfunction (recent myocardial infarction, cardiomyopathies)
      B. Mitral stenosis
      C. Fluid overload
  II. Increased pulmonary capillary permeability (noncardiogenic)
      A. Gram-negative sepsis
      B. Gastric fluid aspiration
      C. Massive transfusion
      D. Blunt chest trauma
      E. Pneumonia
      F. Anaphylaxis
      G. Smoke inhalation
      H. Toxic chemical inhalation
      I. Oxygen toxicity
      J. Fat embolism

    K. Uremia
    L. Near-drowning
    M. Pancreatitis
    N. Post–cardiopulmonary bypass
III. Other
    A. High altitude
    B. Narcotic overdose
    C. Neurogenic
    D. Postobstructive

DISCUSSION

The mechanisms behind pulmonary edema can be understood by studying the Starling law of capillary-interstitial fluid exchange:

$$\text{Fluid accumulation} = K[(P_c - P_{if}) - \sigma(\pi_{pl} - \pi_{if})] - Q_{lymph}$$

where K = permeability coefficient
P_c = mean intracapillary pressure
P_{if} = mean interstitial fluid pressure
σ = reflection coefficient of macromolecules
π_{pl} = oncotic pressure of plasma proteins
π_{if} = oncotic pressure of interstitial fluid
Q_{lymph} = lymphatic flow

The forces that tend to promote fluid movement out of the blood vessels are P_c and π_{if}; these forces are usually offset by π_{pl} and P_{if}, the factors that help retain fluid in the vascular tree. If any fluid does escape, it is removed by the lymphatic system, so overall there is no net accumulation of fluid in the interstitium.

In most cases of cardiogenic pulmonary edema, P_c is greatly increased, the lymphatics are overwhelmed, and fluid accumulates in the lungs. The most common cause is left ventricular (LV) dysfunction due to myocardial infarctions or cardiomyopathies. Pressure in the pulmonary capillaries may increase in the presence of normal LV function when patients have significant mitral stenosis; occasionally, pulmonary edema is the initial manifestation. Massive fluid overload is the third possibility. Not only is P_c increased, but π_{pl} (primarily albumin, a major force in keeping fluid in the intravascular space) is decreased. The net effect is pulmonary edema in patients with normal LV function. Hypoalbuminemic states, without increases in hydrostatic pressure, will not produce pulmonary edema.

In cases of noncardiogenic pulmonary edema (also referred to as the adult respiratory distress syndrome, or ARDS), the Starling principle does not apply. The primary problem is disruption of the alveolar-capillary membrane, with leakage of proteins and fluid into the alveolar space. A large number of different insults can produce ARDS. Gram-negative sepsis, acid aspiration, and massive transfusion are the most common causes. Smoke or toxic chemical inhalation is usually apparent from the patient's history. Oxygen toxicity can contribute to ARDS in as little as 24 hours in patients requiring high inspired oxygen concentrations. The fat embolism syndrome may develop within 72 hours following skeletal trauma to long bones. Neutral fats deposited in the lungs are degraded by serum lipases to free fatty acids that directly produce the lung injury. Other findings include fever, petechiae on the upper chest and axilla, and mental status changes. Near-drowning leads to pulmonary edema due to (1) acid aspiration or (2) hyperosmolar saltwater drawing fluid into the lungs from the vascular space.

Other causes, not related to hemodynamic or capillary membrane changes, are high altitude, narcotic overdose, neurogenic, and postobstructive. Neurogenic pulmonary edema follows central nervous system injury; it is felt to be secondary to massive sympathetic discharge, which produces peripheral vasoconstriction and subsequent hypertension and elevation of central circulating blood volume. Postobstructive pulmonary edema is thought to be due to large negative intrapleural pressures, which produce interstitial edema. The mechanisms behind high-altitude and narcotic overdose pulmonary edema remain obscure.

Laboratory studies are minimally helpful in the diagnosis of pulmonary edema. Arterial blood gases reveal hypoxemia due to intrapulmonary shunts. Interstitial and alveolar edema may be seen on chest radiographs. If the cause is unclear from the history, a pulmonary artery (PA) catheter should be placed to aid in the diagnosis. Cardiogenic pulmonary edema is associated with elevated PA pressures and depressed cardiac output. Noncardiogenic pulmonary edema may have low to normal PA pressures and normal to elevated cardiac output. Echocardiography may be beneficial in quantitating LV function and ruling out mitral stenosis.

SELECTED READING

Allen S: Pathophysiology of pulmonary edema: Implications for clinical management. *39th Annual Refresher Course Lectures and Clinical Update Program.* American Society of Anesthesiologists. Lecture 222, pp 1–6.

Murray TR, Marshall BE: Causes and management of perioperative pulmonary edema. *ASA Refresher Courses Anesthesiol* 15 : 149, 1987.

II
Cardiovascular

13
Intraoperative Hypotension

DEFINITION

Hypotension, one of the most common problems encountered in clinical anesthesia, is defined as a decrease in blood pressure (BP) greater than 20 percent below baseline values. A number of factors contribute to the generation of blood pressure:

1. Blood pressure is the product of total peripheral resistance (TPR) and cardiac output (C.O.):

$$BP = TPR \times C.O.$$

2. Cardiac output is the product of heart rate (HR) and stroke volume (SV):

$$C.O. = HR \times SV$$

3. Therefore,

$$BP = TPR \times HR \times SV$$

4. Stroke volume is determined by interactions of preload, afterload, and cardiac contractility. Once spurious causes have been excluded, decreases in blood pressure must be due to alterations in one of five variables: (1) **TPR**, (2) heart rate or rhythm, (3) ventricular preload, (4) ventricular afterload, and (5) cardiac contractility.

ETIOLOGY

I. Spurious causes
   A. Blood pressure cuff too large
   B. Blood pressure cuff loosely applied
   C. Arterial line problems (improperly zeroed, poorly calibrated, excessively damped)
   D. Peripheral vasoconstriction (hypothermia, alpha-agonist drugs)
II. Decreased total peripheral resistance
   A. Vasodilating drugs
      1. Volatile anesthetics (isoflurane)
      2. Antihypertensive medication (sodium nitro-prusside, hydralazine)
      3. Alpha-adrenergic receptor blockers (droperidol)
   B. Regional anesthesia (subarachnoid or epidural blockade)
   C. Release of aortic cross clamp
   D. Spinal shock
   E. Autonomic neuropathy (diabetic, alcoholic, Guillain-Barré syndrome)
   F. Removal of pheochromocytoma
   G. Carcinoid tumor (serotonin, kinins)
   H. Deliberate hypotension
   I. Altered baroreceptor function
   J. Adrenal insufficiency (Addison's disease, corti-costeroid withdrawal)
III. Changes in heart rate/rhythm
   A. Sinus bradycardia
      1. Drugs (beta-blocking agents, calcium channel blockers, digitalis, anticholinesterase compounds)
      2. Vagal stimulation (oculocardiac reflex, succinyl-choline)
      3. Hypoxia
      4. Sick sinus syndrome
      5. Increased intracranial pressure
      6. Altered baroreceptor function

B. Junctional bradycardia
C. Sinus tachycardia
D. Heart block (second degree type II, third degree)
E. Tachyarrhythmias (paroxysmal atrial tachycardia)
IV. Decreased ventricular preload
  A. Decreased intravascular volume
    1. Acute hemorrhage
    2. Dehydration (vomiting, nasogastric suction, diarrhea, diabetes insipidus, bowel preparation, prolonged NPO status)
    3. Osmotic diuresis (glucose, mannitol)
    4. Third-space fluid losses (peritonitis, trauma)
  B. Decreased venous return
    1. Drugs
      a. Histamine release (morphine, meperidine, vancomycin, d-tubocurarine)
      b. Direct vasodilators (nitrates)
      c. Alpha-adrenergic blockade (droperidol)
    2. Positive-pressure ventilation
    3. Patient position (sitting, reverse Trendelenburg)
    4. Cardiac arrhythmias (atrial fibrillation, junctional rhythm)
    5. Vena caval obstruction (gravid uterus, tumor, tense ascites)
    6. Acute pericardial tamponade
    7. Methylmethacrylate
    8. Tension pneumothorax
    9. Celiac plexus block
    10. Regional anesthesia (subarachnoid or epidural blockade)
    11. Massive pulmonary embolism (thrombus, air)
    12. Atrial myxoma
    13. Complement activation (transfusion reaction, protamine reaction, anaphylaxis, septic shock)
    14. Right ventricular failure (infarctions, pulmonary hypertension)

V. Increased ventricular afterload
  A. Aortic stenosis
  B. Idiopathic hypertrophic subaortic stenosis (IHSS)
  C. Malfunctioning prosthetic heart valve
  D. Vasoconstrictors (phenylephrine)
  E. Placement of aortic cross clamp
VI. Altered cardiac contractility
  A. Cardiac disorders
    1. Myocardial ischemia
    2. Myocardial infarction
    3. Cardiomyopathy (dilated, postpartum)
  B. Drugs
    1. Volatile anesthetic agents (halothane)
    2. Beta-blocking drugs (propranolol)
    3. Calcium entry blockers (verapamil)
    4. Barbiturates (sodium pentothal)
    5. Local anesthetic toxicity (bupivacaine)
  C. Methylmethacrylate
  D. Hypocalcemia

DISCUSSION

Maintenance of normotension is most important in patients with atherosclerotic cardiovascular disease, renal insufficiency, increased intracranial pressure, and pregnancy. The absolute level of blood pressure is important when signs and symptoms of inadequate tissue perfusion develop, primarily altered mentation, angina pectoris, nausea, decreased urine output, and fetal bradycardia or late decelerations. Laboratory studies may reveal lactic acidosis, electrocardiographic (ECG) changes associated with myocardial ischemia, and a decrease in the mixed venous oxygen saturation. Fetal scalp sampling may show a decrease in pH secondary to inadequate placental perfusion.

Initially, spurious causes of hypotension should be excluded (see Chaps. 55 and 59). Sphygmomanometer cuffs that are either too large or not placed snugly on the extremity will give falsely low readings; for pressures to be accurate, the cuff should be approximately two-thirds the width of the extremity circumference. Arterial catheters may record falsely low readings if the transducer (1) is placed too high above the heart, (2) is calibrated incorrectly, or (3) is dampened by air bubbles in the tubing. With either technique, the peripheral pressure may be low while central pressures are near normal if excessive vasoconstriction secondary to hypothermia or alpha-adrenergic agonists exists.

Probably the most frequent cause of intraoperative hypotension is decreased ventricular preload secondary to a decrease in either intravascular volume or venous return. Decreased intravascular volume occurs in acute hemorrhage when blood or crystalloid replacement is inadequate. Dehydration can develop following protracted vomiting, nasogastric suctioning, diarrhea, or uncontrolled diabetes insipidus. In a normal-sized, normothermic adult, dehydration will develop at an average of 100 ml/hour for every 1 hour NPO. Osmotic diuresis secondary to either hyperglycemia or mannitol administration can lead to volume depletion. Third-space fluid losses can produce total body fluid overload in the presence of intravascular hypovolemia; it occurs with highly traumatized tissues, peritonitis, or ascites.

Since two-thirds of the blood volume is normally found in the venous system, factors that decrease venous return will have a profound impact on the stroke volume and ultimately the blood pressure. These factors either (1) increase venous capacitance or (2) decrease blood return to the heart. Medications that increase venous capacitance include vasodilators (nitroglycerin), alpha-adrenergic receptor blockers (droperidol), and nonimmunologic histamine-releasing drugs (morphine, d-tubocurarine, vancomycin). Methylmethacrylate, an agent used to cement prosthetic joints, can precipitate hypotension; while the exact mechanism is unclear, it probably relates to increased venous capacitance and decreased myocardial contractility. Regional anesthesia, including celiac plexus blockade, will precipitate (1) venodilation and a drop in the preload and (2) a decrease in the total peripheral resistance. Anaphylactic reactions induce complement activation, which triggers release of biologically active compounds, including histamine and anaphylatoxins. These agents cause vasodilation and fluid loss due to increased capillary permeability.

In some patients, the volume of the venous system may be normal but cannot return to the left ventricle. Gravitational forces impair venous return when patients are in either the reverse Trendelenburg or sitting position. Vena caval obstruction due to tense ascites or a gravid uterus will block venous return; 10 percent of pregnant women will experience the aortocaval syndrome with hypotension when placed in the supine position without hip tilt. Mechanical ventilation and tension pneumothorax impede venous return, since both cause compression of large thoracic veins. A massive pulmonary embolus will block blood flow from the right to the left ventricle. Right ventricular (RV) failure, secondary to either RV infarction or prolonged pulmonary hypertension, leads to impaired forward flow to the left ventricle. Atrial systole, or the "atrial kick," may contribute up to 40 percent of the left ventricular preload; it is lost with atrial fibrillation and junctional rhythms, leading to a decrease in cardiac output and blood pressure.

The second major cause of hypotension is decreased TPR. While all volatile anesthetic agents decrease TPR, isoflurane is the most potent. Antihypertensive medication, such as sodium nitroprusside, used for deliberate hypotension, and hydralazine are direct vasodilators. Droperidol and phentolamine decrease TPR through alpha-adrenergic blockade.

Multiple physiologic or pathologic processes will cause a decline in the TPR. TPR abruptly decreases following release of an aortic cross clamp, removal of a pheochromocytoma, or development of spinal shock after cervical or high thoracic spinal cord lesion. Patients with long-standing diabetes mellitus or alcoholism can develop autonomic neuropathy, which causes a gradual loss of sympathetic tone. Adrenal insufficiency, primarily due to an abrupt withdrawal of exogenous corticosteroids, can cause profound hypotension when the physiologic stress of surgery is encountered.

Baroreceptors, located in the walls of the internal carotid arteries and aortic arch, play an integral role in rapidly maintaining arterial blood pressure. Activation of the baroreceptor reflex by an elevation in blood pressure produces (1) inhibition of the vasomotor center in the medulla, resulting in vasodilation and (2) stimulation of the vagal center, leading to decreases in heart rate. With hypotension, the opposite reactions occur, causing the pressure to return to normal. Therefore, abnormalities in the baroreceptor reflex can lead to unexpected hypo- or hypertension, which is especially pronounced following a carotid endarterectomy. In sick preterm neonates, the baroreceptor reflex is abolished under general anesthesia; that is, the heart rate does not increase in response to a decrease in blood pressure. Volatile anesthetics, particularly halothane but also isoflurane to a lesser extent, inhibit the heart rate portion of the reflex.

While a decrease in the TPR can directly produce hypotension, an increase in TPR or afterload can lead to hypotension by decreasing either forward blood flow or myocardial function. Aortic stenosis, IHSS, or a malfunctioning prosthetic heart valve can obstruct blood flow from the heart. An acute increase in afterload, as occurs when an aortic cross clamp is placed or when vasoconstrictors such as phenylephrine are administered, can cause hypertension, which can precipitate decreased ventricular function and ultimately hypotension from myocardial failure.

In addition, altered cardiac contractility can develop secondary to intrinsic cardiac disorders or drugs. Both myocardial ischemia and infarction decrease ventricular function, which leads to a decrease in cardiac output. Ischemia and infarction may be detected by (1) ST segment changes on the ECG or (2) wall motion abnormalities on two-dimensional transesophageal echocardiography. Dilated or postpartum cardiomyopathies are usually diagnosed preoperatively; these patients have characteristic symptoms of dyspnea, orthopnea, and paroxysmal nocturnal dyspnea.

A variety of drugs directly depress myocardial performance. Of the volatile anesthetic agents, halothane is the most potent myocardial depressant; intravenous agents such as sodium pentothal can also depress cardiac function. Ketamine causes direct myocardial depression when the patient has exhausted catecholamine stores. Local anesthetic toxicity secondary to intravascular injection of bupivacaine will cause myocardial failure that is often irreversible. Both beta-receptor and calcium entry blocking agents can decrease myocardial function; of the calcium entry blockers, verapamil has the greatest effect. When large quantities of citrate are given with massive blood transfusions, hypocalcemia may develop secondary to calcium chelation by the citrate; however, this condition rarely develops, due to the large calcium stores in the skeleton.

The last general cause of hypotension is alterations in the heart rate or rhythm. Cardiac output may be decreased with sinus bradycardia, since the preload to the left ventricle is decreased. The effect of bradycardia is more profound in infants, since their stroke volume is fixed and cardiac output is directly dependent on heart rate. When bradycardia develops, the most important problem to exclude is hypoxia. The arterial oxygen tension is profoundly depressed before the heart rate decreases; it can usually be detected by pulse oximetry or arterial blood gases. Vagal stimulation directly slows the heart; this response is more pronounced in infants and small children, who have a higher resting vagal tone. It occurs commonly with eye surgery (oculocardiac reflex) or after multiple doses of succinylcholine. Other drugs that can lead to sinus bradycardia include beta-receptor and calcium entry blocking agents and anticholinesterase compounds (edrophonium and neostigmine). Physiologic disorders such as increased intracranial pressure and sick sinus syndrome can cause bradycardia and hypotension.

Other heart rate changes leading to hypotension include tachycardia and various forms of heart block. Tachycardias lead to hypotension by (1) decreased ventricular filling time (sinus tachycardia), (2) loss of "atrial kick" (atrial fibrillation), or (3) myocardial ischemia and impaired contractility due to increased oxygen demand. Both second degree type II and third degree (complete) heart block can lead to hypotension due to a loss of atrial preload and a slow ventricular rate.

If hypotension does not readily respond to initial treatment (administering a fluid bolus, controlling heart rate or rhythm, or decreasing anesthetic concentration) or if the cause of hypotension is unclear, a pulmonary artery (PA) catheter may be needed to provide additional information. With a PA catheter, cardiac output and cardiac filling pressures (central venous pressure [CVP], pulmonary artery occlusion pressure [PAOP]) are directly measured, while the TPR can be calculated using the following equation:

$$TPR = \frac{(MAP - \overline{CVP})}{C.O.} \times 80$$

where $\underline{MAP}$ = mean arterial pressure
$\overline{CVP}$ = mean central venous pressure

The normal values are (1) C.O.: 4 to 7 liters/minute; (2) CVP: 2 to 8 mm Hg; (3) MAP: 60 to 90 mm Hg; (4) PAOP: 6 to 15 mm Hg; and TPR: 900 to 1500 dynes-sec/cm^5. Determining these parameters can aid in diagnosing the cause of intraoperative hypotension. For example, a low cardiac output coupled with decreased filling pressures may be secondary to hypovolemia or decreased venous return, while elevated filling pressures suggest left ventricular failure or cardiac tamponade (Table 13-1). If the cardiac output is elevated while the systemic blood pressure is low, the TPR is usually low; this condition is seen with anaphylactic shock or early stages of septic shock.

Table 13-1. Use of a Pulmonary Artery Catheter in the
Interpretation of Various Low Cardiac Output States

Cause of Low Cardiac Output	CVP	PAo	PAdP vs. PAo Pressure
Hypovolemia	Decreased	Decreased	PAdP = PAo
Left ventricular failure	Increased	Increased	PAdP = PAo
Right ventricular failure	Increased	No change	PAdP = PAo
Pulmonary embolism	Increased	No change	PAdP > PAo
Cardiac tamponade	Increased	Increased	PAdP = PAo

CVP = central venous pressure; PAo = pulmonary artery occlusion pressure;
PAdP = pulmonary artery diastolic pressure.
Source: Stoelting RK, Miller RD: Monitoring. In Stoelting RK, Miller
RD (eds): *Basics of Anesthesia*, 2nd ed. New York: Churchill Livingstone,
1989. P 222.

SELECTED READING

Bashein GT: Cardiac output: Measurement and clinical significance.
41st Annual Refresher Course Lectures and Clinical Update Program.
American Society of Anesthesiologists. Lecture 216, pp 1–7.

Cook PR, Malmqvist LA, Bengtsson M, et al. Vagal and sympathetic
activity during spinal analgesia. *Acta Anaesthesiol Scand* 34 : 271,
1990.

14
Intraoperative Hypertension

DEFINITION

Hypertension is defined as an elevation in the arterial blood pressure. An exact number is difficult to assign, since normal values vary greatly with age; that is, what is normotensive for an adult is usually considered hypertensive in a neonate or child. In general, hypertension in an adult exists when the baseline blood pressure is 140/90 mm Hg or greater, or when the systolic or diastolic pressures are 20 to 30 percent above preoperative values in a previously normotensive patient. Causes of intraoperative hypertension fall into two main categories: (1) preexisting and (2) operative-specific.

ETIOLOGY
I. Preexisting
   A. Essential hypertension
   B. Renal disease (glomerulonephritis, renal artery stenosis, hemolytic-uremic syndrome)
   C. Endocrinopathy (Cushing's disease, pheochromocytoma, hyperaldosteronism)
   D. Coarctation of the aorta
   E. Preeclampsia
   F. Obesity
   G. Tumors (carcinoid, Wilms' tumor)
   H. Increased intracranial pressure (ICP)
II. Operative-specific
   A. Hypoxia
   B. Hypercarbia
   C. Pain

D. Anxiety
E. Inadequate ("light") anesthesia
F. Spurious hypertension (blood pressure cuff too small, errors of intraarterial monitor)
G. Drugs
  1. Withdrawal (antihypertensive medication, alcohol, narcotics)
  2. Anesthetic agents (ketamine, cocaine)
  3. Vasopressors (epinephrine, ephedrine, phenylephrine)
H. Procedure-specific
  1. Aortic cross clamp
  2. Tourniquet pain
  3. Induced hypertension (carotid endarterectomy)
  4. Post–carotid endarterectomy
  5. Cranial nerve stimulation (trigeminal)
I. Hypervolemia (fluids, blood)
J. Autonomic hyperreflexia
K. Bladder distention

DISCUSSION

Hypertension is the most common circulatory disorder affecting patients and is an important risk factor for premature atherosclerotic cardiovascular disease. These patients are at higher risk for perioperative complications, ranging from cerebrovascular accidents and congestive heart failure to myocardial infarction and death. Patients may have preexisting hypertension or hypertension that develops de novo in the operating room. In many cases, the cause of the preexisting hypertension is the reason for the operative procedure, such as removal of a tumor (Wilms', pheochromocytoma, adrenal adenoma), repair of vascular narrowing (coarctation of the aorta, renal artery stenosis), or operative delivery of a fetus (preeclampsia).

In the operating room, the blood pressure may be falsely elevated if (1) the blood pressure cuff is too small for the diameter of the arm or leg, (2) an arterial line is improperly calibrated, (3) the transducer is not positioned properly in relation to the heart, or (4) the resonance in the system is excessive, leading to overshoot. For accurate pressures by cuff, the cuff should be one-third to one-half as wide as the circumference of the extremity (see Chapters 55 and 59).

Overall, the most common form is primary or essential hypertension. Although it accounts for 95 percent of all cases of hypertension, the etiology is unknown. These patients may be on a variety of antihypertensive medications, and abrupt withdrawal of certain drugs preoperatively, such as clonidine or propranolol, can trigger a rebound hypertensive crisis.

Other preexisting disease states that can lead to elevated blood pressure include obesity, renal failure, increased intracranial pressure, and drug or alcohol addiction. Obesity itself may produce hypertension, discounting errors in measurement due to large extremities and inappropriate cuff size. Renal failure leads to hypertension secondary to either the disorder producing uremia, such as glomerulonephritis, or volume overload from inadequate dialysis. In patients with increased ICP, hypertension is a protective mechanism to ensure that cerebral perfusion pressure is maintained; hypertension may resolve with measures that decrease ICP. Patients addicted to alcohol or narcotics may experience rebound hypertension from abrupt drug withdrawal, while illicit drugs, such as amphetamines or cocaine, may directly produce hypertension following ingestion.

At the induction of anesthesia, adequate oxygenation and ventilation should be ensured, since hypoxia and hypercarbia will cause hypertension. Induction agents such as ketamine trigger sympathetic stimulation leading to hypertension and tachycardia. Drugs used for topical anesthesia may directly increase blood pressure (cocaine) or may contain epinephrine; the effects of these drugs are usually transient. Inadequate anesthesia for the degree of stimulation (direct laryngoscopy, skin incision, sternotomy) is probably the most common cause of hypertension and usually resolves with administering additional anesthetic agents; it should be suspected if a patient either moves or is tearing. Inadequate anesthesia is also a stimulus for autonomic hyperreflexia, a condition that develops in patients with spinal cord lesions at T6 or higher or with other cord lesions such as multiple sclerosis. In these cases, the most potent stimulus is distention of a hollow organ, as occurs during cystoscopy. This stimulus leads to a sudden discharge of sympathetic nerves below the level of the cord lesion, which are not under control from higher inhibitory centers. Treatment includes deepening the level of anesthesia or using a specific antihypertensive drug such as sodium nitroprusside.

Several other conditions can produce hypertension in the operating room. Anxiety or pain may lead to mild elevations in blood pressure. Bladder distention can cause hypertension in patients with or without spinal cord lesions. Tourniquet pain produces gradual increases in blood pressure starting about 60 minutes after the cuff is inflated. Hypertension uniformly develops when the aorta is cross clamped for reconstructive surgery. Stimulation of the fifth cranial nerve (trigeminal) during intracranial surgery will manifest as hypertension and bradycardia. During a carotid endarterectomy, hypertension is intentionally created through the use of vasopressors, such as phenylephrine, to enhance perfusion to the brain through collateral vessels.

SELECTED READING

Charlson ME, MacKenzie CR, Gold JP, et al: Preoperative characteristics predicting intraoperative hypotension and hypertension among hypertensives and diabetics undergoing noncardiac surgery. *Ann Surg* 212 : 69, 1990.

Matthews DM, Miller ED: Mechanisms and treatment of perioperative hypertension. *ASA Refresher Courses Anesthesiol* 18 : 237, 1990.

15
Sinus Tachycardia
Raeford E. Brown, Jr., and Roberta E. Galford

DEFINITION

Sinus tachycardia is defined as a heart rate greater than 100 beats per minute (BPM) in an adult and 120 to 140 BPM in a child. The rate is consistent and regular, with impulse formation in the sinoatrial (SA) node and normal conduction through the atrioventricular (AV) node to the ventricles. Since sinus tachycardia is a symptom, not an independent rhythm disturbance, one should search for an underlying cause. Causes of sinus tachycardia fall into four general categories: (1) drugs, (2) drug withdrawal, (3) disease states, and (4) miscellaneous factors.

ETIOLOGY
I. Drugs
   A. Catecholamines (epinephrine, dopamine, cocaine)
   B. Anticholinergics (atropine, glycopyrrolate)
   C. Muscle relaxants (pancuronium, succinylcholine, gallamine)
   D. Vasodilators (sodium nitroprusside, nitroglycerin)
   E. Anesthetic agents (isoflurane, enflurane)
   F. Antidepressants (monoamine oxidase inhibitors, tricyclic antidepressants)
   G. Methylxanthines (aminophylline, caffeine)
   H. Beta-agonists (terbutaline, ritodrine)
   I. Nicotine

II. Drug withdrawal
   A. Alcohol
   B. Narcotics (cocaine, heroin)
   C. Beta-adrenergic blocking agents (propranolol)
   D. Clonidine
III. Disease states
   A. Myocardial ischemia/infarction
   B. Congestive heart failure
   C. Fever
   D. Malignant hyperthermia
   E. Pheochromocytoma
   F. Thyrotoxicosis
   G. Venous air embolism
   H. Anemia
   I. Hypovolemia
   J. Hypoxemia
   K. Hypercarbia
IV. Miscellaneous factors
   A. Anxiety
   B. Pain
   C. Inadequate level of anesthesia
   D. Exercise

DISCUSSION

When evaluating a patient with a heart rate greater than 100 BPM, one should first determine whether the rhythm is of sinus origin or not. With sinus tachycardia, the P waves (1) are upright in leads II, III, and aVF, (2) have a uniform morphology, and (3) will precede each QRS complex. Rarely will the rate be greater than 160 BPM in an adult. When vagal maneuvers (carotid sinus massage, Valsalva) are performed, the rate will gradually slow; when the maneuver is terminated, the rate will gradually return to the previous level. Next, one should look for evidence of myocardial ischemia, since heart rate is a major determinant of myocardial oxygen consumption. If ischemia is present, the heart rate should be slowed while causes of sinus tachycardia are explored.

A review of the patient's history, physical examination, laboratory studies, and medication record often reveal the cause of sinus tachycardia. A patient may be experiencing anxiety or pain; administration of sedatives or narcotics may be beneficial in decreasing the heart rate. The patient may have a history of congestive heart failure (CHF), coronary artery disease, thyrotoxicosis, or substance abuse. The abrupt discontinuance of alcohol or narcotics may precipitate acute withdrawal, with sinus tachycardia developing secondary to sympathetic overactivity. In addition to an elevated heart rate, the vital signs may show orthostatic hypotension, indicative of intravascular volume depletion, tachypnea secondary to respiratory insufficiency, or fever. On physical examination, bibasilar rales or dependent pitting edema signifies uncontrolled CHF while exophthalmos suggests thyrotoxicosis. Laboratory studies may disclose arterial hypoxemia or hypercarbia, anemia, or electrocardiographic (ECG) changes consistent with myocardial ischemia or infarction. The medication record may show a variety of drugs that can increase the heart rate, such as beta-agonists (terbutaline, ritodrine), theophylline compounds, antidepressants, vasodilators, or inotropic drugs, especially dopamine. In addition, inadvertent medication withdrawal (beta-blockers or clonidine, for example) may be discovered.

During the operative procedure, the most common cause of sinus tachycardia is an inadequate level of anesthesia for the degree of surgical stimulation. A significant rise in heart rate at the time of intubation, skin incision, or sternotomy indicates a need to increase the depth of anesthesia. Continuous measurement of oxygen saturation and end-tidal carbon dioxide effectively eliminates hypoxemia and hypercarbia as causative factors. Hypovolemia or anemia may be indicated by hypotension, marked variation in arterial waveform tracing with positive-pressure ventilation, poor peripheral perfusion, and decreased urine output. Myocardial ischemia may be both a cause and an effect of sinus tachycardia; ST segment trend analysis should be performed on a patient with a history of coronary artery disease and an elevated heart rate.

Many anesthetic agents produce sinus tachycardia as a side effect. Both isoflurane and enflurane can lead to sinus tachycardia, although the response is variable. Pancuronium is vagolytic, while succinylcholine produces tachycardia through ganglionic stimulation. Anticholinergics, such as atropine or glycopyrrolate, lead to tachycardia; these agents are given for their antisialagogue effect preoperatively or to combat bradycardia secondary to anticholinesterase medications postoperatively.

Several disease states can trigger sinus tachycardia. Both malignant hyperthermia and thyrotoxicosis produce a hypermetabolic state that leads to increased oxygen demands and ultimately sinus tachycardia. An elevated carbon dioxide level, in the absence of known thyroid disease, should raise the suspicion of malignant hyperthermia. Fever secondary to an infectious process leads to sinus tachycardia, with the heart rate increasing 10 BPM for every 1°F rise in temperature. A pheochromocytoma usually presents with paroxysmal elevations in blood pressure and heart rate. Venous air embolism, a potential complication with sitting surgical procedures, can be diagnosed by monitoring end-tidal nitrogen levels, precordial Doppler, or cardiac echocardiography.

SELECTED READING

Springman SR, Atlee JL: The etiology of intraoperative arrhythmias. *Anesthesiol Clin North Am* 7 : 293, 1989.
Stevenson RL, Rogers MC: Diagnosis of cardiac dysrhythmias. *ASA Refresher Courses Anesthesiol* 14 : 217, 1986.

16
Sinus Bradycardia

Daniel J. Kennedy and Roberta E. Galford

DEFINITION

Sinus bradycardia is defined as a heart rate less than 60 beats per minute (BPM) in an adult and less than 100 BPM in an infant. Sinus bradycardia implies that the controlling pacemaker mechanism originates in the sinus node and that there is a normal, regular relationship between sinus node activity (P wave) and the ventricular response it generates (QRS complex). Although sinus bradycardia may be a normal finding in a young, well-conditioned athlete, it usually is secondary to (1) drug effects, (2) vagal maneuvers, or (3) disease processes.

ETIOLOGY

I. Drug effects
   A. Beta-adrenergic receptor blocking agents (propranolol)
   B. Narcotics (fentanyl, sufentanil)
   C. Calcium entry blocking agents (verapamil)
   D. Digoxin
   E. Potent inhalational agents (halothane)
   F. Antiarrhythmic medication (quinidine, amiodarone)
   G. Anticholinesterase agents (edrophonium, neostigmine)
   H. Succinylcholine
   I. Cholinergic agents (pilocarpine, methacholine)
II. Vagal maneuvers
   A. Oculocardiac reflex
   B. Carotid sinus manipulation

    C. Reflex stimulation (nasopharynx, traction on peritoneum or testicle, distention of hollow viscus)

    D. Reflex bradycardia (increased intracranial pressure, hypertension)

    E. High subarachnoid or epidural block

III. Disease processes

    A. Hypoxia

    B. Myocardial infarction/ischemia

    C. Sinus node disease (sick sinus syndrome, sinus node pause)

    D. Hypothyroidism (myxedema)

    E. Hypothermia

DISCUSSION

The rate of sinus node discharge reflects the balance of sympathetic and parasympathetic input to the heart. Sympathetic input is via the cardiac accelerator fibers, which arise from the stellate ganglion and the cervical sympathetic trunk, while parasympathetic input is via the vagus nerve; normally, parasympathetic tone predominates. Circulating mediators, such as cholinergic agents or catecholamines, may act directly on receptors for these systems or may exert their effect by stimulating autonomic ganglia.

    Although there are many causes of sinus bradycardia in an anesthetic setting, hypoxia should always be considered first. For bradycardia to be secondary to hypoxia, the oxygen saturation must be profoundly depressed. Supplemental oxygen should be administered while arterial blood gases or pulse oximetry is being measured. Second, the patient's hemodynamic status should be closely monitored. Slow heart rates may be tolerated in well-trained athletes if the blood pressure and cardiac output are maintained at normal levels; in other individuals, particularly in the elderly, bradycardia may lead to hypotension, presyncope, or impaired mentation. Pediatric patients, primarily infants, are especially sensitive to sinus bradycardia; in these patients, cardiac output is directly dependent on heart rate since their stroke volume is fixed. Third, heart rates less than 35 to 40 BPM increase the risk of an escape focus firing and may give rise to ectopic beats and possibly more serious rhythm disturbances.

Drugs are the most common cause of sinus bradycardia; they may slow the sinus rate either directly or indirectly. Beta-blockers diminish the effect of cardiac accelerator fibers input at the receptor level, while verapamil and similar calcium entry blockers directly decrease output from the sinus node. Anticholinesterase compounds, such as edrophonium and neostigmine, cause an increase in acetylcholine at the neuromuscular junction and a subsequent increase in muscarinic receptor stimulation, leading to bradycardia; cholinergic agents, such as methacholine, have a similar effect. Potent inhalation agents (primarily halothane) and narcotics (except meperidine) can produce decreases in heart rate. Bradycardia secondary to halothane administration is most likely due to decreases in sympathetic tone, while fentanyl leads to central vagal stimulation. The combination of fentanyl and vecuronium has been reported to produce severe bradycardia and even asystole. Digoxin is an uncommon cause of sinus bradycardia. Other drugs that can lead to sinus bradycardia include antiarrhythmic medications, such as quinidine and amiodarone.

Succinylcholine may lead to bradycardia in children with the first dose and in adults with doses repeated every 5 to 10 minutes. It is thought that succinylcholine, by virtue of its acetylcholine-like activity, stimulates nicotinic receptors in the autonomic ganglia and muscarinic receptors in the sinus node; the latter effect is blocked by prior atropine administration. The phenomenon of bradycardia with successive doses of succinylcholine in adults is not well understood. However, it may be related to byproducts of succinylcholine hydrolysis (succinylmonocholine, choline), which may sensitize the heart to subsequent doses.

Vagal maneuvers are the second major cause of bradycardia. Pressure on the eye or traction on the extraocular muscles triggers the oculocardiac reflex, which is especially pronounced in children. Manipulation of the carotid sinus during a carotid endarterectomy can cause a decrease in heart rate that is blocked by topical administration of local anesthetics on the carotid sinus itself. Intraoperative traction on the peritoneum or testicles can cause vagally mediated slowing of the heart rate, even in patients with adequate regional anesthesia, since the vagus nerve is not affected by subarachnoid or epidural blockade. Bradycardia secondary to vagal stimulation usually resolves with cessation of the surgical manipulation.

Reflex bradycardia can develop secondary to profound hypertension; in these cases, sympathetic tone is inhibited secondary to baroreceptor stimulation in the carotid sinus. It can occur when the afterload of the heart is acutely increased, as when the aorta is cross clamped or when a vasoconstrictor such as phenylephrine is administered. Increased intracranial pressure, by virtue of compression of autonomic centers in the brainstem, can lead to the Cushing response, a triad consisting of hypertension, bradycardia, and respiratory irregularities. Bradycardia secondary to increased intracranial pressure is an ominous finding.

Several disease states can lead to sinus bradycardia. In the elderly, disease of the sinus node can lead to sinus arrest, sinus pause, and sick sinus syndrome. Myocardial ischemia or infarction may lead to profound bradycardia or heart block, particularly when the right coronary artery is involved. Hypothyroidism may be undiagnosed at the time of surgery and should be considered as an uncommon cause of bradycardia. Hypothermia may contribute to bradycardia by virtue of a generalized slowing of metabolism.

SELECTED READING

Doyle DJ, Mark PW: Reflex bradycardia during surgery. *Can J Anaesth* 37 : 219, 1990.
Kerr CR, Grant AO, Wenger TL, Strauss HC: Sinus node dysfunction *Cardiol Clin* 1 : 187, 1983.

17
ST Segment Alterations

DEFINITION

The ST segment is the portion of the electrocardiogram (ECG) extending from the end of the QRS complex, called the J point, to the beginning of the T wave. The normal ST segment is (1) straight or slightly convex downward and (2) isoelectric, although there may be slight elevation or depression around the baseline. To be considered normal, the elevation should be less than 1 mm and depression less than 0.5 mm; changes from baseline greater than this amount usually indicate significant pathology. Changes in the ST segment in one ECG lead often cause reciprocal alterations in the opposite leads. Causes of ST segment elevation or depression fall into two general categories: (1) cardiac causes and (2) noncardiac causes.

ETIOLOGY

I. ST segment elevation
   A. Cardiac causes
      1. Myocardial infarction/injury
      2. Prinzmetal's angina
      3. Acute pericarditis
      4. Left ventricular hypertrophy (LVH) (V_1)
      5. Hypertrophic cardiomyopathy
      6. Left bundle branch block (LBBB) (V_1)
   B. Noncardiac causes
      1. Normal variant (early repolarization)
      2. Hyperkalemia
      3. Cerebrovascular accident (subarachnoid hemorrhage)

4. Profound hypothermia (<30°C)
5. Metastatic carcinoma to the heart
6. Acute cor pulmonale

II. ST segment depression
  A. Cardiac causes
    1. Myocardial ischemia
    2. Subendocardial infarction
    3. Left ventricular hypertrophy (V_6)
    4. Right ventricular hypertrophy (RVH)
    5. Left bundle branch block (V_5–V_6)
    6. Right bundle branch block (V_1–V_2) (RBBB)
    7. Permanent ventricular pacemaker
  B. Noncardiac causes
    1. Electrolyte disturbances
      a. Hypokalemia
      b. Hypercalcemia
    2. Drugs
      a. Digitalis
      b. Class I antiarrhythmics (quinidine)
      c. Phenothiazines
      d. Emetine

DISCUSSION

The ST segment and T wave represent phases 2 and 3 of the cardiac action potential, when ventricular repolarization occurs. Repolarization, a more diverse process than depolarization, takes longer and proceeds in a nonuniform pattern; therefore, ST segment abnormalities, with or without T wave changes, are commonly seen. Up to 10 percent of all ECGs will have the reading of "nonspecific ST–T wave changes." However, significant elevation or depression of the ST segment indicates an underlying cardiac or noncardiac disturbance.

ST segment elevation is classically seen in myocardial infarction (MI), Prinzmetal's (vasospastic) angina, and acute pericarditis. In both infarction and Prinzmetal's angina, the altered ST segments correlate with the diseased coronary artery (II, III, and aVF—right coronary; V_1 to V_4—left anterior descending; V_5 and V_6—left circumflex). Historical findings of acute exertional chest pain associated with diaphoresis, nausea, and vomiting are found in an acute MI, while Prinzmetal's angina, by definition, occurs at rest. In contrast, the ST segment changes of acute pericarditis are diffuse, occurring over various leads. Pleuritic chest pain is usually present, and on auscultation of the chest a pericardial friction rub may be heard. Other cardiac causes of ST segment elevation in lead V_1 include LVH and LBBB.

A variety of noncardiac conditions can produce ST segment elevation (Fig. 17-1). A normal variant, called "early repolarization," can occur in young black males, with ST segment elevation up to 4 mm in the precordial leads. Acute cor pulmonale secondary to pulmonary embolism may produce ECG changes resembling an inferior wall MI; if the pulmonary embolism is massive, an RBBB pattern may develop. Profound hypothermia (body temperature below 30°C) can cause an elevation of the J point; this configuration is referred to as an Osborne wave (Fig. 17-2). Hyperkalemia, with a serum potassium level greater than 6.0 mEq/liter, will produce tall, peaked T waves and ST segment elevation; as the potassium level further increases, the ECG assumes a sine wave appearance. Other noncardiac causes include cerebrovascular accidents, primarily subarachnoid hemorrhage, and metastatic carcinoma to the heart.

ST segment depression can indicate a number of cardiac disorders. Both myocardial ischemia and subendocardial myocardial infarction will have ST depression in the leads representing the involved artery. A patient who has sustained a subendocardial MI may later have a normal ECG without characteristic Q waves that develop following a transmural infarction. Bundle branch blocks cause downward deflections of the ST segment, which appear in leads V_1 and V_2 with RBBB and V_5 and V_6 with LBBB pattern. A permanent

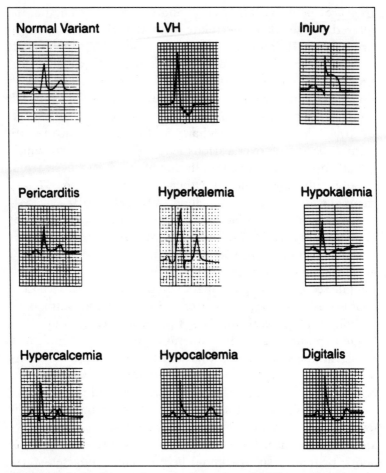

Figure 17-1. Cardiac and noncardiac causes of ST segment changes. (From McAnulty J: Electrocardiography. In JH Stein [ed]: *Internal Medicine*, 3rd ed. Boston: Little, Brown 1990. P. 35.)

ventricular pacemaker produces a pattern similar to LBBB, while LVH with strain and RVH also show ST segment depression. When LBBB or LVH with strain is present, myocardial ischemia cannot be diagnosed on the basis of an ECG.

Electrolyte disturbances and drug effects account for the noncardiac causes of ST segment depression. Hypokalemia

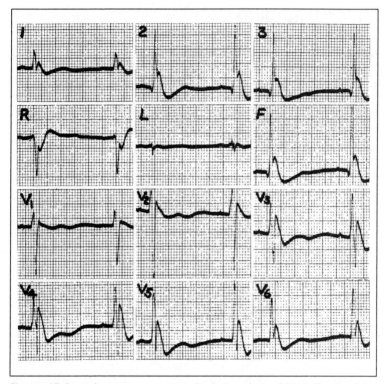

Figure 17-2. Osborne waves—marked elevation of "J deflection" characteristic of profound hypothermia. (From Marriott HJL: *Practical Electrocardiography.* © 1977, the Williams & Wilkins Co., Baltimore.)

leads to ST segment depression, flattened T waves, and when severe, the development of U waves. Hypercalcemia routinely shortens the Q–T interval and occasionally depresses the ST segment. The classic example of drug-induced changes is produced by digitalis, which affects the lateral precordial leads; ST segment depression alone does not indicate digitalis toxicity. Both phenothiazines and quinidine produce changes indistinguishable from hypokalemia. A rare cause of ST segment depression is emetine, a compound used for the treatment of amebiasis.

SELECTED READING

Clements FM, deBruijn NP: Detection of myocardial ischemia and infarction. *Anesthesiol Clin North Am* 6 : 545, 1988.

Kohli RS, Cashman PM, Lahiri A, Raftery EB: The ST segment of the ambulatory electrocardiogram in a normal population. *Br Heart J* 60 : 4, 1988.

18
Cardiac Arrest/ Electromechanical Dissociation

DEFINITION

Cardiac arrest is defined as an antemortem, potentially reversible state of cardiac standstill. It is usually due to an arrhythmia, primarily ventricular tachycardia (VT), ventricular fibrillation (VF), profound sinus bradycardia, or asystole. Electromechanical dissociation (EMD) is the absence of effective mechanical action of the heart, with normal organized electrical activity on the electrocardiogram (ECG). Sudden death is defined as an unexpected, nontraumatic fatality occurring in patients with or without preexisting disease who die within 6 hours of the onset of the terminal event. Although extensive atherosclerotic coronary artery disease is the most common cause of all three, a variety of other, often reversible, processes can lead to either cardiac arrest or EMD.

ETIOLOGY
I. Cardiac arrest
  A. Cardiac disorders
    1. Myocardial infarction
    2. Myocardial ischemia
    3. Cardiomyopathy (congestive, hypertrophic)
    4. Valvular heart disease
    5. Congenital Q–T syndrome
    6. Primary electrical heart disease (preexcitation syndrome, sick sinus syndrome)

B. Electrolyte disturbances
  1. Hypokalemia
  2. Hyperkalemia (potassium chloride, succinyl-choline)
  3. Hypomagnesemia
C. Hypoxia
D. Acidosis
E. Trauma
  1. Cardiac contusion
  2. Cardiac tamponade
  3. Tension pneumothorax
  4. Aortic dissection
F. Drugs
  1. Tricyclic antidepressant overdose
  2. Cocaine
  3. Class I antiarrhythmics (quinidine, procainamide)
  4. Digitalis toxicity
  5. Methylxanthines
  6. Sympathomimetic drugs
  7. Phenothiazines
G. Drowning or near-drowning
H. Electrocution
I. Hypothermia
II. Electromechanical dissociation
  A. Correctable causes
    1. Acute hypovolemia
    2. Cardiac tamponade
    3. Tension pneumothorax
    4. Hypoxia
    5. Acidosis
    6. Shock (anaphylactic, neurogenic, septic)
  B. Less correctable causes
    1. Massive myocardial infarction
    2. Prolonged myocardial ischemia
    3. Pulmonary embolism

DISCUSSION

Many of the same pathologic processes can produce either cardiac arrest or EMD. Myocardial infarction (MI) or ischemia accounts for up to 50 percent of out-of-hospital cardiac arrests, with evidence of infarction seen in 25 percent of the survivors. In the remaining cases, other cardiac disease (valvular heart disease, sick sinus syndrome, prolonged Q–T interval, cardiomyopathy) is the underlying cause; for example, cardiac arrest in young, healthy male athletes is often due to idiopathic hypertrophic subaortic stenosis (IHSS). Often the underlying disease process is so extensive that the patient cannot be resuscitated; when EMD occurs in the presence of an acute MI, the prognosis is poor due to the massive amount of tissue damage.

Trauma is the most common cause of cardiac arrest or EMD in young individuals. Significant trauma can lead to EMD secondary to hypovolemia, cardiac tamponade, or tension pneumothorax. Hypovolemic shock should be suspected when external blood loss is profuse or if the neck veins are flat when a patient is supine. Cardiac tamponade can occur after (1) a deceleration injury due to the impact of a steering wheel or (2) a stab wound to the chest or upper abdomen. A tension pneumothorax can develop after penetrating injury to the thorax; it may become apparent after positive-pressure ventilation via an endotracheal tube. Other causes of shock, such as sepsis, anaphylaxis, or neurogenic disorders, can lead to EMD. Acute hypoxia or acidosis may be a major contributor to EMD in trauma victims. In addition, these individuals may have taken drugs, such as cocaine or amphetamines, which can lead to cardiac arrest.

Hypothermia, electrocution, and drowning or near-drowning are special causes of cardiac arrest. When the patient's core temperature drops to less than 32°C, the heart is extremely irritable; even simply moving the patient can trigger ventricular fibrillation that is unresponsive to cardioactive drugs.

With profound hypothermia, reflex vasoconstriction makes detection of peripheral pulses difficult; a person may appear to be clinically dead but is still viable if aggressive management is immediately instituted. Alcohol ingestion increases the risk of hypothermia by (1) causing peripheral vasodilation, which promotes heat loss and (2) impairing an awareness of the environment.

Drowning leads to profound hypoxia and acidosis, occasionally in the absence of aspiration. Drowning may be complicated by hypothermia; cold water immersion accelerates heat loss, since the thermal conductivity of water is 32 times greater than air. The dangers of accidental electrocution are related to the duration and magnitude of the electrical current. While low-voltage arrests happen at home, the majority of high-voltage arrests occur in the workplace.

Many drugs can produce cardiac arrhythmias. Cocaine precipitates a massive sympathetic discharge which leads to ventricular fibrillation. Hypoxia and acidosis following cocaine-induced seizures can contribute to the arrhythmogenic potential of the drug. Methylxanthine toxicity (theophylline) or sympathomimetic drugs can also cause marked sympathetic stimulation. Toxicity from antiarrhythmic medications may actually generate more malignant rhythm disturbances. Digitalis toxicity can lead to various arrhythmias that are exacerbated by hypokalemia. The class I antiarrhythmic agents quinidine and procainamide can cause a prolongation of the Q–T interval leading to polymorphic ventricular tachycardia or torsades de pointes (see Chap. 22).

Acute electrolyte disturbances can induce ventricular arrhythmias. Hypomagnesemia can cause VT that is refractory to antiarrhythmic medication unless the magnesium level is corrected. Hyperkalemia, due to intravenous administration of potassium or acute potassium release from muscle depolarization triggered by succinylcholine, can precipitate VT or VF. Hypokalemia alone or in the presence of digitalis can lead to arrhythmias.

SELECTED READING

Caplan RA, Ward RJ, Posner K, Cheney FW: Unexpected cardiac arrest during spinal anesthesia: A closed claim analysis of predisposing factors. *Anesthesiology* 68 : 5, 1988.

Olsson GL, Hallén B: Cardiac arrest during anaesthesia: A computer-aided study in 250,543 anaesthetics. *Acta Anaesthesiol Scand* 32 : 653, 1988.

19
Wide Complex Tachycardia

DEFINITION

Wide complex tachycardia is defined as a ventricular rate greater than 100 beats per minute (BPM) with a QRS complex duration greater than 0.12 second. The origin of the tachycardia is either (1) supraventricular with abnormal conduction or (2) ventricular.

ETIOLOGY
  I. Supraventricular tachycardia (SVT)
     A. With aberrancy
     B. With preexisting bundle branch block
 II. Ventricular
     A. Ventricular tachycardia (VT)
     B. Torsades de pointes
     C. Ventricular preexcitation syndromes
     D. Ventricular flutter/fibrillation
     E. Ventricular paced rhythms

DISCUSSION

The characterization of wide complex tachycardia (WCT) should begin after evaluation of the patient's hemodynamic stability. Many of these rhythms result in low cardiac output, hypotension, or pulselessness; synchronized cardioversion or defibrillation may be necessary prior to definitive diagnosis. Only when the patient is stable should attempts to delineate the etiology of the tachycardia be undertaken. The most common cause of WCT is VT, especially in patients with underlying heart disease (coronary artery disease, cardiomyopathy, left ventricular hypertrophy). Therefore, if the diagnosis is unclear, the patient should be treated for presumed VT.

Distinguishing SVT with abnormal conduction from VT is often difficult. If discrete atrial activity is not apparent, other criteria are used to distinguish between the two groups (Table 19-1). The most reliable criterion for VT is finding atrioventricular (AV) dissociation. AV dissociation is defined as the independent beating of the atria and ventricles so that P waves, indicative of atrial activity, can be found embedded in the QRS complex. It occurs in up to 50 percent of cases of VT; when present, it confirms that the abnormal beats are of ventricular origin (Fig. 19-1).

Other criteria, though less definitive but which support the diagnosis of VT, include (1) heart rate of 130 to 170 BPM, (2) QRS duration greater than 0.14 second in the absence of pre-existing bundle branch block or drugs that widen the QRS complex (quinidine, procainamide), (3) presence of fusion

Table 19-1. Ventricular Versus Supraventricular Tachycardia

Characteristic	Ventricular	Supraventricular
QRS width	> 0.14 second	< 0.14 second
Heart rate	130–170 BPM	> 170 BPM
AV dissociation	Frequent	Uncommon
Fusion beats	Diagnostic	Absent
PACs normally conducted	Yes	No
Other	Capture beats	Ashman's phenomenon (see Chap. 20)
	Marked left axis deviation	

AV = atrioventricular; PACs = premature atrial contractions.

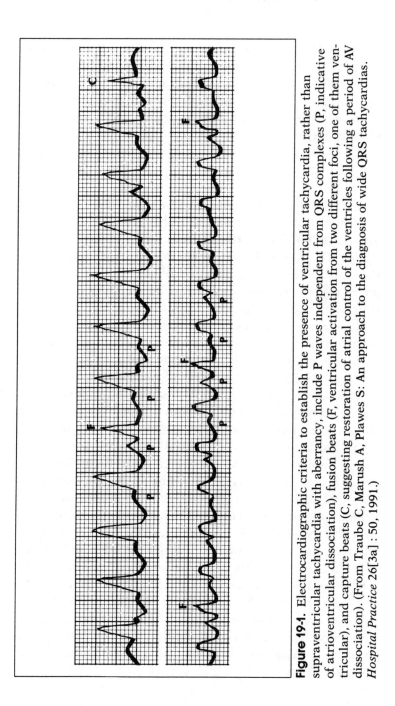

Figure 19-1. Electrocardiographic criteria to establish the presence of ventricular tachycardia, rather than supraventricular tachycardia with aberrancy, include P waves independent from QRS complexes (P, indicative of atrioventricular dissociation), fusion beats (F, ventricular activation from two different foci, one of them ventricular), and capture beats (C, suggesting restoration of atrial control of the ventricles following a period of AV dissociation). (From Traube C, Marush A, Plawes S: An approach to the diagnosis of wide QRS tachycardias. *Hospital Practice* 26[3a] : 50, 1991.)

beats, or (4) premature atrial contractions (PACs) that are normally conducted prior to the onset of the WCT. Fusion beats occur when the ventricles are activated by two simultaneous impulses, one descending from the atria and one arising from the ventricles; the electrocardiogram (ECG) shows intermittent narrowing of the QRS complex. When a fusion beat is seen in the midst of a WCT, it indicates that the tachycardia is ventricular in origin. Lastly, although VT is often described as very regular, it may initially be irregular.

Several other ventricular rhythms can cause WCT. Pre-excitation syndromes, such as Wolff-Parkinson-White, may give rise to WCT with extremely rapid ventricular rates (up to 300 BPM). The classic delta wave may or may not be seen on the resting ECG before the onset of the WCT. A ventricular paced rhythm is usually evident from a history of a permanent ventricular pacemaker plus the appearance of pacer spikes on the surface ECG. Ventricular fibrillation is characterized by chaotic, disorganized electrical activity that may be coarse or fine. Since no discrete mechanical activity is present, it is associated with no appreciable cardiac output and pulselessness; it requires immediate defibrillation.

A frequent cause of WCT is SVT with abnormal ventricular conduction. The supraventricular rhythm may be sinus tachycardia, paroxysmal SVT, atrial tachycardia with block, atrial fibrillation, atrial flutter, or accelerated junctional tachycardia. There may be (1) a preexisting bundle branch block, (2) a block that presents only at accelerated rates, called a rate-dependent bundle branch block, or (3) conditions that can cause the QRS complex to widen, such as hyperkalemia, cardiomyopathy, or drugs. Atrial fibrillation is described as irregularly irregular, while any regular rhythm with a ventricular response near 150 BPM should raise the possibility of atrial flutter with 2 : 1 AV conduction. Paroxysmal supraventricular tachycardia often occurs in young individuals without underlying cardiac disease, while atrial tachycardia with block is virtually diagnostic of digitalis toxicity (see Chap. 20).

SELECTED READING

Herschman Z, Kaufman B: Differential diagnosis of wide complex tachycardias. *Anesthesiol Clin North Am* 7 : 351, 1989.

Stewart RB, Bardy GH, Greene HL: Wide complex tachycardia: Misdiagnosis and outcome after emergent therapy. *Ann Intern Med* 104 : 766, 1986.

20
Narrow Complex Tachycardia

DEFINITION

A narrow complex tachycardia (NCT) is defined as a heart rate greater than 100 beats per minute (BPM) in an adult with a QRS complex duration less than 0.12 second. The narrow QRS complex implies a normal electrical activation sequence through the atrioventricular (AV) node, conducting system, and ventricles. Although in rare instances the rhythm arises from the ventricles, the vast majority is supraventricular in origin.

ETIOLOGY
   I. Sinus tachycardia (see Chap. 15)
  II. Paroxysmal supraventricular tachycardia (PSVT)
 III. Atrial tachycardia with block
  IV. Multifocal atrial tachycardia
   V. Atrial flutter
  VI. Atrial fibrillation
 VII. Preexcitation syndrome

DISCUSSION

When a patient presents with a NCT, one should first ensure the patient's hemodynamic stability. Rapid heart rates may lead to increased myocardial oxygen consumption, resulting in myocardial ischemia and decreased cardiac output. If hypotension or cerebral or myocardial hypoperfusion is present, treatment with beta-adrenergic blockers, such as esmolol, or synchronized cardioversion may be indicated before diagnostic evaluation.

The most common form of NCT, sinus tachycardia, is discussed in Chapter 15. The remaining NCTs can be characterized by (1) the underlying abnormality leading to the tachycardia (enhanced automaticity versus circus movement) or (2) clinical presentation (paroxysmal versus nonparoxysmal). Enhanced automaticity occurs when an irritable focus develops in the atria or AV node, while circus movements are secondary to reentry in either the atria or the AV node. With either mechanism, the P wave is abnormal while the QRS complex is normal. Paroxysmal describes sudden onset (and usually offset), while nonparoxysmal implies a gradual onset; determining whether the onset is paroxysmal is helpful in diagnosing the rhythm disturbance.

PSVT is the term applied to rhythms previously referred to as paroxysmal atrial tachycardia (PAT) or paroxysmal junctional tachycardia. PSVT often occurs in healthy young people without preexisting coronary or valvular heart disease. It is characterized by abrupt onset and termination, with a regular rhythm ranging from 150 to 230 BPM. In contrast, atrial tachycardia with block is almost always due to either digitalis toxicity or underlying cardiac disease. The atrial rate is 150 to 200 BPM with a P wave that is morphologically different from a sinus node-generated P wave. The ventricular rate varies with the degree of AV block.

Atrial fibrillation (AF) is most commonly seen in patients with ischemic or hypertensive heart disease, mitral valve disease, or after open heart surgery secondary to atrial irritation caused by the atriotomy site. Occasionally it develops in healthy individuals, precipitated by the stresses of surgery, anesthesia, or exercise. AF is characterized by the absence of organized atrial activity. AV conduction varies, leading to an "irregularly irregular" rhythm. Aberrant intraventricular conduction of impulses can occur and is referred to as Ashman's phenomenon. In this condition, a relatively long R–R interval is followed by a short R–R interval. The impulse arising after the short interval will often encounter the right bundle in its refractory period; therefore, the impulse is conducted with a right bundle branch block configuration. When a patient is in AF, the arterial line tracing shows marked variation in the blood pressure due to loss of the "atrial kick."

Multifocal atrial tachycardia (MAT) and atrial flutter are discussed in conjunction with atrial fibrillation (AF) since they often degenerate into AF. MAT, by definition, has at least three morphologically different P waves, indicating that it arises from at least three foci. The atrial rate ranges from 100 to 150 BPM, with 1 : 1 AV conduction. The most common cause is underlying pulmonary disease; other causes include potassium and magnesium disturbances, fever, and beta-adrenergic stimulation.

In atrial flutter, the atrial rate is approximately 300 BPM. Since the AV node cannot conduct such rapid rates, varying degrees of AV block develop (2 : 1, 4 : 1). The most common is 2 : 1 AV block, which gives rise to a regular ventricular rate of 150 BPM. A characteristic finding on the electrocardiogram is a sawtooth pattern; it is secondary to flutter waves and is most prominent in leads II, III, and aVF. Atrial flutter rarely occurs in the absence of underlying disease and is most commonly associated with ischemic or valvular heart disease and acute or chronic pulmonary disorders.

Preexcitation syndromes are rare causes of NCT. Wolff-Parkinson-White syndrome occasionally may present with a NCT. Lown, Ganong, and Levin described a syndrome with a normal P–R interval and a narrow QRS complex. It may be precipitated by surgical stresses, anesthesia, or premature atrial contraction.

SELECTED READING

Bar FW, Brugada P, Dassen WR, Wellens HJ: Differential diagnosis of tachycardia with narrow QRS complex (shorter than 0.12 sec). *Am J Cardiol* 54 : 555, 1984.

Chester WL: Differential diagnosis of narrow complex tachycardias. *Anesthesiol Clin North Am* 7 : 337, 1989.

21
Heart Block

Daniel J. Kennedy and Roberta E. Galford

DEFINITION

Heart block is defined as delayed propagation of the electrical impulses through the cardiac conduction system. It is characteristically classified as first degree, second degree (types I and II), and third degree (or complete) heart block. First degree and second degree type I are normally benign and produced by processes that are transient or reversible, while second degree type II and complete heart block indicate significant organic heart disease that usually is not reversible. Causes of heart block can be divided into three major categories: (1) increased vagal tone, (2) decreased sympathetic tone, or (3) atrioventricular (AV) nodal dysfunction.

ETIOLOGY

   I. Increased vagal tone
      A. Physiologic
         1. Carotid sinus manipulation
         2. Distention of hollow viscus
         3. Oculocardiac reflex
         4. Diving reflex
         5. Bezold-Jarisch reflex
      B. Drugs
         1. Cholinergic agents (methacholine)
         2. Anticholinesterase agents (edrophonium, neostigmine)

        3. Narcotics (fentanyl, sufentanil)
        4. Potent inhalational agents (halothane)
        5. Digoxin

II. Decreased sympathetic tone
    A. Physiologic
        1. Hypothermia
        2. Sleep/unconsciousness
    B. Drugs
        1. Beta-adrenergic receptor blocking agents (propranolol)
        2. Central alpha-adrenergic receptor blocking agents (clonidine)
        3. Ganglionic blocking agents (guanethidine)
        4. Narcotics

III. AV nodal dysfunction
    A. Anatomic
        1. Congenital (syphilis, leopard syndrome)
        2. Myocardial infarction
        3. Myocarditis/cardiomyopathy
        4. Degenerative disease (Lenegre's)
        5. Infiltrative diseases (sarcoidosis, scleroderma, gout, hemochromatosis, amyloidosis)
        6. Valvular heart disease (aortic, mitral)
        7. Inflammatory heart disease (rheumatic fever, Reiter's)
        8. Traumatic injury (following cardiac surgery or placement of a pulmonary artery catheter)
        9. Cardiac tumors (mesothelioma, myxoma, lymphoma)
      10. Infectious disease (syphilis, toxoplasmosis, mumps)
    B. Functional
        1. Good physical conditioning (athletes)
        2. Myocardial ischemia
        3. Electrolyte disturbances (hyperkalemia, hypo-magnesemia)
        4. Severe acidosis

5. Mitral valve prolapse syndrome
6. Endocrine disorders (adrenal insufficiency, hyperthyroidism, hypothyroidism)
7. Hypothermia

C. Drugs
1. Calcium entry blocking agents (verapamil)
2. Beta-adrenergic receptor blocking agents
3. Digoxin

DISCUSSION

When evaluating a patient with heart block, the first consideration is to ensure the patient is hemodynamically stable. A
patient may be symptomatic from second degree type I block
or totally asymptomatic from third degree heart block. Symptoms range from altered mentation to syncope secondary to
decreased cerebral perfusion. Secondly, it should be realized
that heart block due to increased vagal tone or decreased sympathetic tone is often transient, while AV nodal dysfunction,
particularly anatomic derangements, is usually permanent.

Heart block most commonly arises from abnormal conduction through the AV node and is classified according to the
degree of AV nodal dysfunction. First degree heart block represents slowed conduction through the proximal AV node and
is defined as a prolonged P–R interval greater than 0.20 second (Fig. 21-1). Each P wave is followed by a QRS complex,
and no QRS complex occurs without a preceding P wave. First
degree block is usually asymptomatic and does not require
treatment. It occurs secondary to drugs, such as digoxin or
beta-blockers, diseases, such as rheumatic heart disease, or
electrolyte disturbances, such as hypomagnesemia. When
drug concentrations are excessive, complete heart block can
be produced but resolves with drug elimination or excretion.

With second degree heart block, some but not all P waves
fail to traverse the AV node and thus do not generate a QRS
complex. Second degree heart block has two types, Mobitz I
and Mobitz II. Mobitz I, also called Wenckebach or proximal

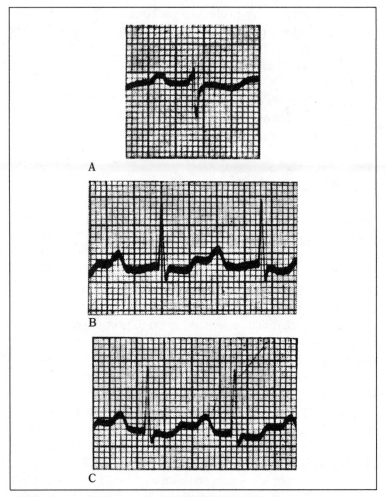

Figure 21-1. First degree AV block with prolonged P–R interval. (From HJL Marriott: *Practical Electrocardiography*. © 1977, the Williams & Wilkins Co., Baltimore.)

block, is characterized by progressive lengthening of the P–R interval until finally one P wave is not conducted and therefore no QRS complex is produced (Fig. 21-2). The cycle then repeats, and the relation of P waves to QRS complexes is

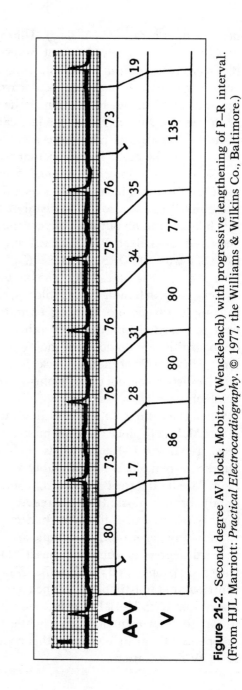

Figure 21-2. Second degree AV block, Mobitz I (Wenckebach) with progressive lengthening of P–R interval. (From HJL Marriott: *Practical Electrocardiography.* © 1977, the Williams & Wilkins Co., Baltimore.)

described as a ratio (3 : 2, 4 : 3). This type of heart block is usually temporary and does not progress to complete heart block. It results from reflex slowing of AV conduction as occurs with carotid massage, oculocardiac reflex (bradycardia or heart block due to traction on the extraocular muscles), or the Bezold-Jarisch reflex; the last can occur with inferior-posterior myocardial infarctions secondary to stimulation of receptors in the posterior ventricular wall. Mobitz I may also develop as a function of heightened vagal tone in well-trained athletes. Proximal heart block is usually atropine-sensitive.

Mobitz II block, also called distal or type II heart block, is much less common but more severe than type I. It is (1) characterized by a fixed P–R interval and (2) classified by the ratio of P waves to QRS complexes (3 : 2, 5 : 4) (Fig. 21-3). This type of block originates below the bundle of His, is frequently associated with bundle branch blocks, and usually progresses to complete heart block. It is seen more often with anterior wall myocardial infarctions or other anatomic disturbance (myocarditis, amyloidosis) of the AV node or conduction system. This form of heart block is atropine-resistant and requires isoproterenol or epinephrine to increase the speed of conduction.

When the ratio is 2 : 1, it is difficult to differentiate Mobitz I from Mobitz II, since there are no successive P–R intervals to measure. If the P–R interval is prolonged and there is no bundle branch block, it is probably Mobitz I, while it is more likely Mobitz II if the P–R is normal and there is an associated bundle branch block. High-degree AV block, a severe form of type II block, exists if fewer than one-half of the P waves successfully generate QRS complexes.

Third degree, or complete, heart block occurs when no P waves are propagated through the AV node and there is either ventricular standstill or an escape focus in the distal conducting system (Fig. 21-4). In the latter case, the atria continue to fire at their own intrinsic rate while the escape focus fires independently at its own rate; this condition is also referred to as AV dissociation.

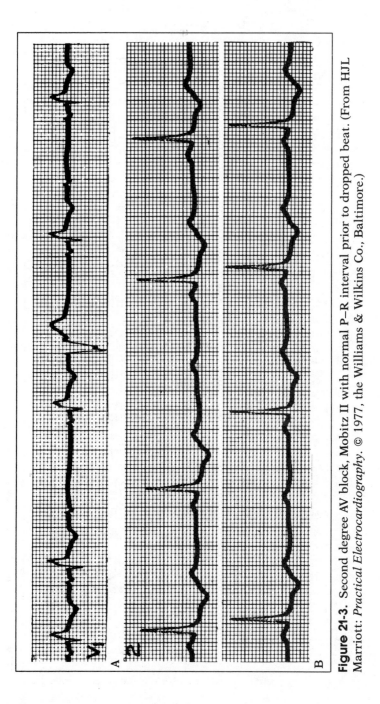

Figure 21-3. Second degree AV block, Mobitz II with normal P–R interval prior to dropped beat. (From HJL Marriott: *Practical Electrocardiography.* © 1977, the Williams & Wilkins Co., Baltimore.)

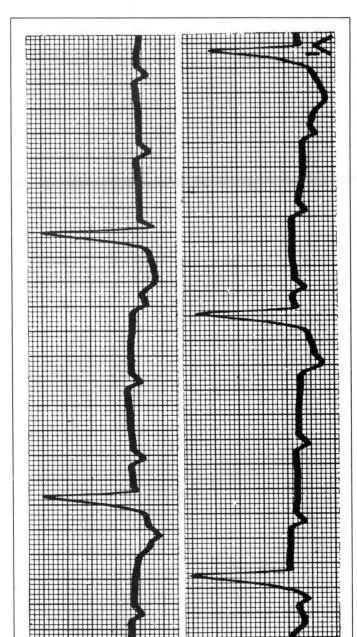

Figure 21-4. Third degree AV block with independent atrial and ventricular activity. (From HJL Marriott: *Practical Electrocardiography.* © 1977, the Williams & Wilkins Co., Baltimore.)

Common causes of complete heart block are Lenegre's and Lev's disease. Lenegre's disease is due to degenerative changes in the conduction system, without involvement of other cardiac tissues; this process is accelerated by chronic hypertension. Lev's disease is secondary to sclerosis and calcification of cardiac structures, such as aortic or mitral valve ring, impinging on fascicles in the conducting system. The end result is interruption of conduction and heart block. It can also occur following cardiac surgery with disruption of tissues adjacent to the mitral anulus. A second iatrogenic cause of complete heart block follows placement of a pulmonary artery catheter in a patient with a preexisting left bundle branch block. It appears to be due to direct trauma to the right bundle, as the risk is increased in patients with right coronary artery disease. In this situation, the heart block may resolve with catheter removal. Otherwise, third-degree heart block requires treatment with a transvenous or transthoracic pacemaker.

SELECTED READING

Puech P, Wainwright RS: Clinical electrophysiology of atrioventricular block. *Cardiol Clin* 1 : 209, 1983.

Ross AF, Martins JB: Recognition and treatment of bradycardias and atrioventricular block. *Anesthesiol Clin North Am* 7 : 373, 1989.

22
Prolonged Q–T Interval

Daniel J. Kennedy and Roberta E. Galford

DEFINITION

The Q–T interval is defined as the time between the onset of the QRS complex and the end of the T wave as measured on the surface electrocardiogram (ECG). The Q–T interval, which correlates with ventricular depolarization and repolarization, is rate-related; as a rough rule, it should compose less than half the length of the total cardiac cycle. Often the Q–T interval is expressed as Q–Tc, where it is "corrected" for heart rate according to the following formula:

$$Q–Tc = Q–T/\sqrt{\text{previous R–R cycle length}}$$

When corrected, the upper limits of normal are 0.39 to 0.46 second for men and 0.44 to 0.47 second for women. Prolongation of the Q–T interval can be either congenital or acquired, with the latter caused by primary cardiac disorders or systemic effects of diseases or drugs on cardiac conduction.

ETIOLOGY
I. Congenital prolongation
   A. Sporadic
   B. Romano-Ward syndrome
   C. Jervell and Lange-Nielsen syndrome
II. Acquired prolongation
   A. Primary cardiac disease states
      1. Myocardial ischemia

  2. Myocardial infarction
  3. Congestive heart failure
  4. Myocarditis
  5. Rheumatic fever
  6. Mitral valve prolapse syndrome
 B. Noncardiac disease states
  1. Cerebrovascular disease (subarachnoid hemorrhage)
  2. Hypothermia
  3. Drastic weight loss (liquid protein diet)
 C. Drug effects
  1. Class Ia antiarrhythmic agents (procainamide, quinidine, disopyramide)
  2. Class Ic antiarrhythmic agents (encainide, flecainide, propafenone)
  3. Other antiarrhythmic agents (amiodarone, bretylium)
  4. Psychotropic drugs (phenothiazines, lithium, tricyclic antidepressant agents)
 D. Electrolyte disturbances
  1. Hypocalcemia
  2. Hypomagnesemia
  3. Hypokalemia

DISCUSSION

Prolongation of the Q–T interval is problematic, since it predisposes patients to cardiac arrhythmias. Premature ventricular contractions and ventricular tachycardia (VT) frequently occur when the Q–T interval is prolonged. A specialized form of VT, torsades de pointes, is characterized by a wide-complex tachycardia, where the QRS complex constantly changes amplitude and morphology such that it appears to be rotating or twisting around the baseline (Fig. 22-1). This rhythm is often unresponsive to standard medical treatment; in fact, many of the drugs used to treat VT, such as procainamide or

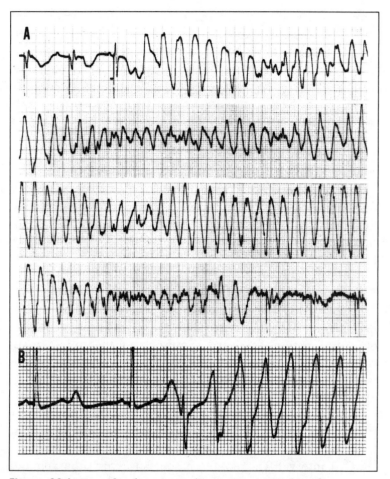

Figure 22-1. Torsades de pointes. (From Zipes DP: Specific arrhythmias. In E Braunwald [ed]: *Heart Disease. A Textbook of Cardiovascular Medicine*, Vol. 1, 3rd ed., Philadephia: W.B. Saunders, 1988. P 699.)

quinidine, may aggravate the arrhythmia by further widening the Q–T interval.

The Q–T interval may be prolonged by two genetically transmitted disorders. Romano-Ward syndrome is autosomal dominant while Jervell and Lange-Nielsen syndrome is autosomal recessive; the latter is associated with congenital nerve deafness. These disorders appear to produce imbalanced sympathetic input to the ventricles; this imbalance may lead to different repolarization rates within the ventricle, predisposing to arrhythmias. Increased sympathetic activity may worsen the Q–T prolongation in these cases and exacerbate the arrhythmias. Patients with congenital prolongation may benefit from beta-adrenergic blockade or other methods to decrease sympathetic tone, such as sympathectomy or stellate ganglion interruption; circumstances that increase sympathetic tone either directly (epinephrine) or indirectly (ephedrine) should be avoided. In contrast, the acquired forms of Q–T prolongation are treated by increasing sympathetic tone, since increasing heart rate will shorten the refractory period and ultimately the Q–T interval.

Acquired Q–T prolongation associated with cardiac disease states reflects a disturbance in repolarization due to (1) inadequate oxygen delivery to sustain high-energy bond generation needed for repolarization (myocardial ischemia or infarction) or (2) dysfunction of the cardiac muscle cells themselves (myocarditis, congestive heart failure, rheumatic fever). Mitral valve prolapse may be associated with Q–T prolongation, although the exact mechanism is not well understood.

Several noncardiac disease states can produce Q–T prolongation. Intracerebral diseases may alter autonomic output from the central nervous system, which leads to increases in the Q–T interval. The most common causes are subarachnoid hemorrhage and intracranial tumors. Hypothermia is associated with generalized slowing of metabolism in cardiac muscle cells and conduction tissue; a reduction in the generation and regeneration of high-energy stores leads to delayed repolarization. The pathophysiology leading to prolongation of the Q–T interval seen with starvation secondary to liquid protein diets is poorly understood.

Drugs can prolong the Q–T interval through a variety of mechanisms. The class Ia antiarrhythmic agents block fast sodium channels, which leads to slowing of the conduction velocity and prolonging of the effective refractory period; class Ic agents have a similar mechanism. In contrast, amiodarone blocks fast sodium channels that have already been opened, thereby preventing their closure. Tricyclic antidepressants and phenothiazines, particularly thioridazine, also decrease cardiac conduction velocity.

Electrolyte disturbances affect the myocyte's ability to generate and maintain cellular membrane potentials; thus, conduction through cells with these altered membrane potentials may be either slowed or blocked altogether. Hypomagnesemia and hypocalcemia are the most common electrolyte disturbances producing a prolonged Q–T interval. Hypocalcemia may develop secondary to massive blood transfusion, although the effect on the Q–T interval is transient due to rapid calcium mobilization from bone. Hypokalemia, although frequently cited as a cause, produces Q–T prolongation only when hypocalcemia is present.

SELECTED READING

Benhorin J, Merri M, Alberti M, et al: Long QT syndrome: New electrocardiographic characteristics. *Circulation* 82 : 521, 1990.

Torline RL, Samuelson PN: Arrhythmias common to infants and children. *Anesthesiol Clin North Am* 7 : 401, 1989.

23
Pulmonary Hypertension

DEFINITION

Pulmonary hypertension is defined as pulmonary vascular pressure greater than 20 mm Hg. It is not a disease but a hemodynamic abnormality secondary to a variety of disorders. Causes of pulmonary hypertension are classified based on the site of primary injury as (1) precapillary or (2) postcapillary.

ETIOLOGY

I. Precapillary
  A. Vasoconstriction
    1. Parenchymal lung disease (chronic bronchitis, emphysema, cystic fibrosis)
    2. Restrictive chest wall disease (kyphoscoliosis)
    3. Neuromuscular diseases (poliomyelitis, myasthenia gravis)
    4. Persistent fetal circulation
    5. High-altitude disease
    6. Central respiratory disorders (primary central hypoventilation, obesity-hypoventilation [pickwickian] syndrome)
  B. Anatomic reduction of the vascular bed
    1. Primary pulmonary hypertension
    2. Recurrent pulmonary thromboembolism
    3. Congenital heart disease (ventricular septal defect, atrial septal defect)
    4. Pulmonary vasculitis (scleroderma)

5. Peripheral pulmonary artery stenosis
6. Diffuse lung disease (adult respiratory distress syndrome [ARDS], interstitial pulmonary fibrosis)
7. Lung resection (lobectomy, pneumonectomy)
8. Schistosomiasis
9. Kyphoscoliosis
II. Postcapillary
   A. Left ventricular failure
   B. Mitral valve disease (stenosis, regurgitation)
   C. Left atrial myxoma
   D. Left atrial thrombus
   E. Veno-occlusive disease
   F. Congenital heart disease (cor triatriatum, pulmonary vein stenosis)

DISCUSSION

Normally, the pulmonary vascular bed is a low-resistance, high-flow circuit; the entire cardiac output perfuses the lungs each minute at one-fifth the mean systemic pressure (12 ± 2 mm Hg) and at one-twelfth the systemic vascular resistance (SVR). Any disorder that increases pulmonary vascular resistance (PVR) will lead to an elevation in pressure. The essential factor in these disorders is a decrease in the cross-sectional area of the pulmonary vascular bed, which leads to increases in PVR. The persistent pressure overload facing the right ventricle ultimately produces right-sided heart failure; *cor pulmonale* is the term applied to right ventricular failure in the absence of ischemic, congenital, or valvular heart disease.

The pulmonary vasculature can be affected by either pre-capillary or postcapillary processes. Postcapillary disorders (left ventricular failure, mitral valve disease) initially produce pulmonary venous hypertension with pressures up to 25 to 30 mm Hg. The presenting symptoms, characteristic of congestive heart failure, include dyspnea, orthopnea, and paroxysmal nocturnal dyspnea (PND). The chest radiograph reveals prominence of the upper lobe veins and Kerley B lines.

For pulmonary blood flow to be maintained, pulmonary artery (PA) pressures must rise; this condition is termed passive pulmonary hypertension, since the gradient across the vascular bed usually remains normal (6 ± 2 mm Hg) and the mean PA pressure rarely exceeds 35 to 40 mm Hg. The exception is long-standing mitral stenosis, where the gradient may exceed 12 mm Hg. An uncommon disorder in children or young adults is veno-occlusive disease. It is characterized by diffuse fibrous narrowing or obliteration of the veins and venules, leading to a picture similar to primary pulmonary hypertension. It is usually fatal within 2 years. Other rare causes of postcapillary PA hypertension include left atrial myxoma or thrombus and some forms of congenital heart disease (cor triatriatum).

With precapillary pulmonary hypertension, the PA pressure increases (mean greater than 20 mm Hg) while the pulmonary capillary wedge and left atrial pressures remain normal (less than 12 mm Hg); therefore, the gradient across the pulmonary circuit exceeds 12 mm Hg. These patients are dyspneic but do not experience orthopnea or PND. The chest radiograph may show right ventricular enlargement and prominent pulmonary arteries, while the left ventricle is normal and Kerley B lines are absent.

Precapillary pulmonary hypertension results from one of two pathologic mechanisms: (1) vasoconstriction or (2) anatomic reduction of the pulmonary vascular bed. Vasoconstriction, which increases PVR, is primarily due to hypoxia or acidosis. Hypoxia is the most potent stimulus acting directly on pulmonary arteries and arterioles. Acidosis interacts synergistically with hypoxia to increase PVR, while alkalosis decreases the pressor response to hypoxia. Infants with persistent fetal circulation (PFC) have vasculature that is highly reactive to hypoxia and acidosis. The effect of alkalosis on the pulmonary vessels is the reason for administering sodium bicarbonate to infants with PFC. Causes of alveolar hypoxia (high-altitude disease, chronic bronchitis, emphysema) or alveolar hypoventilation (neuromuscular diseases, kyphoscoliosis, central respiratory disorders) will lead to hypoxemia, hypercapnia, elevated PVR, and ultimately pulmonary hypertension.

The secondary mechanism producing precapillary pulmonary hypertension is anatomic reduction in the pulmonary vascular bed. This reduction may be due to surgery (lung resection), vasculitis (scleroderma), diffuse lung disease (ARDS or interstitial pulmonary fibrosis) or congenital heart disease. Interstitial pulmonary fibrosis may be secondary to sarcoidosis, radiation fibrosis, or pulmonary asbestosis; when the cause is unknown, it is termed idiopathic pulmonary fibrosis. Long-standing congenital heart lesions with left-to-right shunts such as a ventricular septal defect or less often an atrial septal defect, produce chronic overload to the pulmonary circuit, which leads to hypertrophy of the arteriolar muscle. When hypertrophy develops, the PA pressures remain elevated, the PVR becomes fixed, and the shunt may reverse direction. It is called the Eisenmenger reaction, a condition that may not be reversible with surgical correction of the septal defect. Lastly, patients with severe kyphoscoliosis may have both an anatomic reduction in the vascular bed and vasoconstriction secondary to alveolar hypoxia, producing pulmonary hypertension.

One of the most common causes of precapillary pulmonary hypertension is recurrent pulmonary emboli, with occlusion of the pulmonary vessels ensuing over months. It is associated with alveolar hyperventilation and profound elevation in the PA pressures, similar to primary pulmonary hypertension. In contrast, primary pulmonary hypertension is the rarest cause of elevated PA pressures. It is a disease of unknown origin, developing in the absence of intrinsic cardiac or pulmonary disease. It occurs three to four times more often in women than men. It is diagnosed by pulmonary angiography and cardiac catheterization, which reveals marked elevation in right-sided pressures with low to normal left-sided pressures.

It is important to determine the exact mechanism creating pulmonary hypertension. Passive pulmonary hypertension usually can be reversed by treating left ventricular failure or by replacing the mitral valve. An increase in PVR secondary to vasomotor mechanisms may be attenuated, if not reversed, with correction of hypoxia and acidosis. However, when the increased PVR is fixed, little can be done to correct it except a heart-lung transplant.

SELECTED READING

Hawkins JW, Dunn MI: Primary pulmonary hypertension in adults. *Clin Cardiol* 13 : 382, 1990.

Rasch DK: Pulmonary hypertension. In *Decision Making in Anesthesiology*. Toronto: Decker, 1987. Pp 210–211.

24
Changes in Mixed Venous Oxygen Saturation

Daniel J. Kennedy and Roberta E. Galford

DEFINITION

Mixed venous oxygen saturation ($S\bar{v}O_2$) is defined as the percentage of hemoglobin saturated with oxygen in the right ventricle or pulmonary artery. It represents a mixture of blood that has traversed the arterial system and is returning to the heart via the great vessels, and reflects the balance between oxygen demand and oxygen supply for the body as a whole. A normal value is 65 to 80 percent, with a venous oxygen tension of 35 to 40 mm Hg. Both increases and decreases in the $S\bar{v}O_2$ can indicate significant pathology.

ETIOLOGY
I. Increased $S\bar{v}O_2$
   A. Left-to-right shunts (peripheral, intracardiac)
   B. Hyperdynamic states (sepsis, cirrhosis)
   C. Cellular poisoning (cyanide toxicity)
   D. Decreased oxygen consumption (general anesthesia, hypothermia)
   E. High arterial oxygen tension (high fractional inspired oxygen concentration)
   F. Technical malfunction (wedged catheter, improper calibration, air in blood sample)
   G. Shift in oxyhemoglobin dissociation curve to the left

> H. "Arterialization" of blood sample
> I. Severe mitral regurgitation
II. Decreased $S\bar{v}O_2$
>> A. Low cardiac output states (cardiogenic shock, hypovolemic shock, aortic insufficiency, late septic shock)
>> B. Increased oxygen consumption (fever, shivering, seizures)
>> C. Decreased oxygen delivery (anemia, arterial hypoxemia)
>> D. Shift of oxyhemoglobin dissociation curve to the right

DISCUSSION

Blood samples are drawn from the right ventricle or proximal pulmonary artery (PA) via a PA catheter to measure $S\bar{v}O_2$; measurements from blood collected from central venous catheters in the superior or inferior vena cava are often inaccurate because of differences in oxygen consumption between the upper and lower body. When samples are collected, the balloon should be deflated and the initial 2.5 ml of blood should be discarded, since it represents dead space in the PA catheter. If the sample is drawn too vigorously, pulmonary capillary blood may be collected, giving a falsely elevated $S\bar{v}O_2$; this condition is referred to as arterialization of the PA blood sample. In a similar manner, severe mitral regurgitation causes oxygenated blood to course back across the pulmonary circuit. Other technical errors occur when either the syringe contains air or the tip of the catheter is wedged. Some newer PA catheters are capable of continuous saturation monitoring using fiberoptic reflectance oximetry.

The $S\bar{v}O_2$ is a mixture of blood that passes through capillary beds where oxygen is extracted, along with the small fraction of blood that bypasses capillaries so oxygen extraction cannot occur. It reflects the global balance between oxygen consumption and supply. In normal individuals, tissue oxygen consumption is independent of oxygen delivery. However, when oxygen demand outstrips supply, normal tissue beds increase oxygen extraction (the exception is the myocardium, where oxygen extraction is maximal at baseline). Certain pathologic states, such as fever, shivering, or seizures, lead to increased oxygen extraction secondary to elevated tissue oxygen consumption. The net result is that the postcapillary venules have a lower oxygen tension and therefore a lower than normal $S\bar{v}O_2$.

In many conditions, the tissue oxygen demand is normal, while the delivery is decreased. The classic example is a low cardiac output state secondary to cardiogenic shock or congestive heart failure. A decreased $S\bar{v}O_2$ is often the first sign of inadequate peripheral perfusion, developing before metabolic acidosis; in fact, it is not until the mixed venous oxygen tension falls to 27 to 30 mm Hg that the serum lactate level increases. Other causes of decreased oxygen delivery include anemia and arterial hypoxemia. A shift to the right of the oxyhemoglobin dissociation curve, secondary to acidosis, hypercapnia, or fever, leads to increased oxygen extraction and a decreased $S\bar{v}O_2$. In general, a decreased $S\bar{v}O_2$ is a measure of tissue oxygen supply.

Increased $S\bar{v}O_2$ occurs either when the oxygen supply exceeds demand or the blood bypasses capillary extraction. This latter condition, called shunting, leads to oxygenated arterial blood mixing directly with venous blood, causing the oxygen tension in the venous blood to increase. Shunts are seen with intracardiac lesions, such as ventricular or atrial septal defects with left-to-right blood flow, surgically created arteriovenous fistula, or diseases such as early sepsis, hepatic cirrhosis, or Osler-Weber-Rendu syndrome. A ventricular septal defect may complicate an anteroseptal myocardial infarction; a step-up in oxygen content between blood collected in the right atrium and right ventricle is diagnostic. Elevated oxygen delivery to the tissues, such as occurs when a patient is receiving an increased inspired oxygen concentration, will increase the arterial oxygen tension and subsequently the $S\bar{v}O_2$. Lastly, the $S\bar{v}O_2$ may increase when tissue utilization is decreased, as can develop with general anesthesia, hypothermia, or cyanide toxicity. Cyanide toxicity will cause an elevated $S\bar{v}O_2$ in association with lactic acidosis.

SELECTED READING

Nelson LD: Continuous venous oximetry in surgical patients. *Ann Surg* 203 : 329, 1986.
Vender J: Mixed venous oximetry and its clinical application. *41st Annual Refresher Course Lectures and Clinical Update Program.* American Society of Anesthesiologists. Lecture 135, pp 1–7.

III
Central Nervous System

25
Seizures

DEFINITION

A seizure is the abrupt alteration in electrical activity of the brain. It may be an isolated episode or recur over weeks to months; the latter condition is termed epilepsy. Seizures may present as sensory, motor, or behavioral events; when motor symptoms predominate, it is referred to as a convulsion. Many different types of seizures exist, with tonic-clonic, or grand mal, being one of the most common. Tonic-clonic seizures may result from a variety of different neurologic or systemic insults.

ETIOLOGY
I. Neurologic
    A. Head trauma (primary brain injury, subdural/epidural hematoma)
    B. Brain tumor
    C. Birth injury
    D. Infection (meningitis, encephalitis, abscess)
    E. Arteriovenous malformation
    F. Cerebrovascular accidents
    G. Idiopathic
II. Systemic
    A. Hypoxia
    B. Metabolic
        1. Hypoglycemia/hyperglycemia
        2. Hyponatremia/hypernatremia
        3. Hypocalcemia/hypercalcemia
        4. Hypomagnesemia

C. Drugs
   1. Drug withdrawal (alcohol, narcotics, barbiturates)
   2. Anticonvulsant drug withdrawal
   3. Cocaine
   4. Anesthetic agents (enflurane, isoflurane, ketamine, etomidate, methohexital, meperidine, local anesthetic toxicity)
D. Febrile seizures
E. Other
   1. Uremia
   2. Hepatic failure
   3. Acute intermittent porphyria
   4. Thyrotoxicosis
   5. Eclampsia
   6. Malignant hyperthermia
   7. Sepsis

DISCUSSION

As tonic-clonic seizures can be life-threatening, treatment and diagnosis often occur simultaneously. The foremost considerations are (1) to maintain a patent airway and (2) to provide adequate ventilation and oxygenation. Muscle relaxants may be needed to facilitate endotracheal intubation. Secondly, the seizure should be terminated; if the seizure is not self-limiting, anticonvulsant drugs, such as sodium pentothal, diazepam, or phenytoin, should be given.

Once the patient is medically stable, the etiology of the seizure must be investigated. Historical findings of importance include history of seizures (epilepsy, anticonvulsant medication withdrawal), birth injury, fever (central nervous system infection, febrile seizures), head trauma (primary brain injury, subdural or epidural hematomas), alcoholism (acute alcohol withdrawal, hepatic failure), drug abuse (cocaine intoxication, narcotic or barbiturate withdrawal), and pregnancy (eclampsia). Recent mental status changes or headaches may indicate a mass lesion, such as a tumor or arteriovenous malformation. Rare causes of seizures include sepsis, renal failure, acute intermittent porphyria, and malignant hyperthermia.

Routine laboratory studies (arterial blood gases, serum electrolytes, calcium, magnesium, glucose) should be obtained to help determine correctable causes of seizures. Correctable biochemical abnormalities include hypoxia, hypo- and hyperglycemia, hypo- and hypernatremia, hypo- and hypercalcemia, and hypomagnesemia. These problems should be rectified and the underlying cause of the metabolic derangement identified. Hypoglycemia can occur in diabetics who received insulin or long-acting oral hypoglycemic agents without adequate exogenous glucose coverage. Hyponatremia is common after transurethral resection of the prostate, particularly if the resection time is greater than one hour. Hypocalcemia can develop after (1) parathyroid adenoma resection or (2) total thyroidectomy if the parathyroid glands were removed. Other diagnostic tests that may be done include electroencephalogram (EEG), computerized tomography (CT), and magnetic resonance imaging (MRI) of the brain.

Certain anesthetic agents may produce seizures or seizure-like activity. Drugs that lower seizure threshold include enflurane (particularly with hypocarbia), methohexital, and ketamine. Meperidine can cause seizures if large doses are given intravenously or if the patient is also receiving monoamine oxidase inhibitors. Local anesthetic toxicity may produce grand mal seizures, especially if injected intra-arterially. Etomidate can cause myoclonus; these involuntary movements may resemble seizures but are not associated with epileptiform discharges on the EEG.

SELECTED READING

Modica PA, Tempelhoff R: Seizures during emergence from anesthesia. *Anesthesiology* 71 : 296, 1989.

Modica PA, Tempelhoff R, White PF: Pro- and anticonvulsant effects of anesthetics (part I). *Anesth Analg* 70 : 303, 1990.

Modica PA, Tempelhoff R, White PF: Pro- and anticonvulsant effects of anesthetics (part II). *Anesth Analg* 70 : 433, 1990.

26
Increased Intracranial Pressure

DEFINITION

Intracranial pressure (ICP) is defined as the pressure within the cranial vault; normal values range from 6 to 14 mm Hg. The contents of the cranial vault can be divided into three compartments: (1) brain, (2) cerebrospinal fluid, and (3) cerebral blood volume. The cranium (or skull) is a rigid structure with a limited volume; the relationship between volume and pressure within it is called intracranial compliance. A small increase in the volume of one compartment will lead to a decrease in volume in one or both of the other compartments, and compliance will be decreased. As volume increases further, compensatory mechanisms are exhausted and ICP increases, producing intracranial hypertension (Fig. 26-1). The causes of increased ICP can be classified according to increases in volume of the specific cranial compartments.

ETIOLOGY
 I. Brain
   A. Mass lesion (tumor, hematoma)
   B. Cerebral edema
   C. Cerebral swelling
 II. Cerebrospinal fluid
   A. Decreased absorption
   B. Increased production (choroid plexus papilloma, enflurane)
   C. Obstructive hydrocephalus

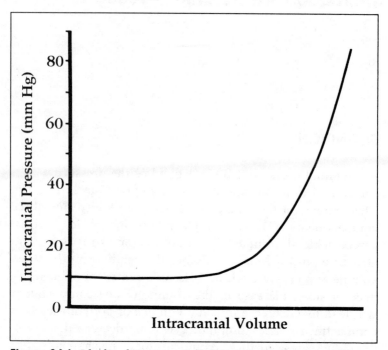

Figure 26-1. Idealized intracranial pressure–volume curve. (From Donegan J: Physiology and metabolism of the brain and spinal cord. In Newfield P, Cottrell JE [eds]: *Neuroanesthesia: Clinical and Physiological Essentials.* Boston: Little, Brown, 1983. P 14.)

III. Cerebral blood volume (or flow)
  A. Hypoxemia
  B. Hypercarbia
  C. Increased mean arterial pressure
  D. Loss of autoregulation (head trauma)
  E. Increased metabolic activity (pain, anxiety, seizures)
  F. Venous outflow obstruction (kinked internal jugular vein central venous catheter)
  G. Anesthetic agents (ketamine, succinylcholine, volatile anesthetics)
  H. Vasodilators (sodium nitroprusside)

I. Sympathetic stimulation (light anesthesia)
J. Trendelenburg's position
K. Increased airway pressure (positive-end expiratory pressure, large tidal volumes)

DISCUSSION

Intracranial pressure (ICP) and mean arterial pressure (MAP), the major determinants of cerebral perfusion pressure (CPP), are related in the following way:

$$CPP = MAP - ICP$$

Any increase in ICP will lead to a decrease in CPP and ultimately to brain ischemia due to inadequate tissue perfusion. Therefore, the major reason to control ICP is to prevent decreases in CPP and ultimately to minimize neuronal damage. Many of the factors that can lead to increased ICP are eliminated by surgical procedures; these procedures include (1) evacuating a hematoma or tumor, (2) shunting obstructive hydrocephalus, or (3) removing a choroid plexus papilloma, a source of CSF overproduction. Other therapeutic interventions fall under the general heading of neuroresuscitative care and are aimed at the factor leading to the ICP elevation.

The first step is to ensure adequate oxygenation and ventilation by frequently monitoring arterial blood gases. Cerebral blood volume (CBV) is directly related to cerebral blood flow (CBF), and factors that affect CBF will ultimately affect CBV. Hypoxemia is the most potent stimulus affecting cerebral blood flow. CBF remains relatively constant when arterial oxygen tension (PaO_2) is greater than 50 mm Hg; however, below this value, CBF increases dramatically. Also, CBF is linearly related to arterial carbon dioxide tension ($PaCO_2$); a 1 mm Hg increase or decrease in $PaCO_2$ leads to a 4 percent change in CBF in the same direction. Therefore, hyperventilation is a major technique to reduce CBF and subsequently ICP (Fig. 26-2).

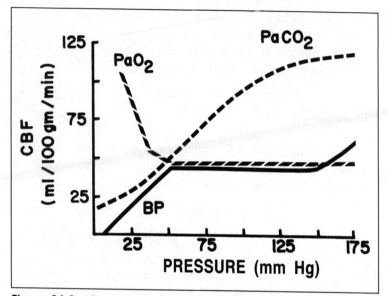

Figure 26-2. Changes in CBF due to alterations in PaCO₂ (*dashed line*), PaO₂ (*parallelogram dashes*), and blood pressure (*solid line*). The other two variables remain stable at normal values when the remaining variable is altered. (From Drummond JC, Shapiro HM: Cerebral Physiology. In Miller RD [ed]: *Anesthesia*, 3rd ed. New York: Churchill Livingstone, 1990. P 625.)

Two other physiologic factors that have a direct impact on CBF are (1) metabolic activity of the brain and (2) MAP. There is a direct coupling of cerebral metabolic requirement for oxygen ($CMRO_2$) and CBF. $CMRO_2$ increases with pain and anxiety and markedly increases with seizures. Intraoperatively, one must maintain a high index of suspicion for seizures, as the paralyzed patient receiving general anesthesia will not exhibit the usual physical manifestations. The second factor is MAP. CBF remains relatively constant over the pressure range of 50 to 150 mm Hg, while it is linearly related to MAP above or below these values. This phenomenon, called autoregulation, is lost with conditions such as head trauma, and CBF becomes directly related to MAP; therefore, as MAP increases, CBF increases.

Certain drugs can affect CBF. Vasodilators, such as sodium nitroprusside, directly increase CBF. Intravenous anesthetic agents, except ketamine, decrease CBF as long as carbon dioxide retention is avoided; with these drugs, $CMRO_2$ and CBF remain coupled. Volatile anesthetics lead to an uncoupling of $CMRO_2$ and CBF, as they increase CBF while decreasing $CMRO_2$. The impact on CBF is greatest with halothane and least with isoflurane and is attenuated for all agents with hyperventilation (Fig. 26-3). In addition, enflurane can contribute to ICP elevation by (1) increasing CSF production and (2) triggering seizure activity exacerbated by hypocarbia.

Head trauma can lead to increased intracranial pressure through a variety of mechanisms. First, it may produce mass lesions such as epidural or subdural hematomas. Second, it can cause either cerebral swelling or cerebral edema. Cerebral swelling is a condition that occurs in children 24 to 48 hours following head trauma; it is due to an increase in cerebral blood flow. In contrast, cerebral edema is an actual increase in brain water content; it develops more commonly in adults. The distinction between cerebral swelling and edema is important since therapeutic interventions will vary.

Nonpharmacologic factors that may increase CBF and subsequently ICP include impaired venous drainage (kinked internal jugular vein, Trendelenburg's position), light anesthesia, and increased airway pressure or positive end-expiratory pressure (PEEP). The effect of positive airway pressure on ICP is unpredictable. It should be remembered, however, that while PEEP may increase ICP, hypoxemia *will* increase ICP.

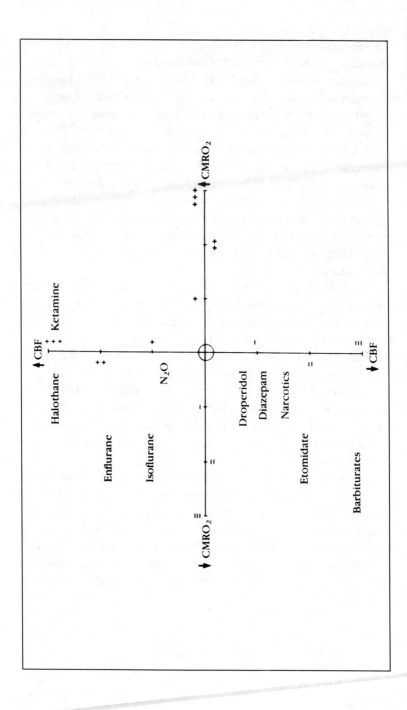

SELECTED READING

Lehman LB: Intracranial pressure monitoring and treatment: A contemporary view. *Ann Emerg Med* 19 : 295, 1990.

Michenfelder J: Cerebral protection and the control of elevated intracranial pressure. *41st Annual Refresher Course Lectures and Clinical Update Program.* American Society of Anesthesiologists. Lecture 115, pp 1–4.

Figure 26-3. Effect of anesthetic agents on the relationship between cerebral blood flow (CBF) and metabolism ($CMRO_2$). Increases and decreases in CBF are indicated along the vertical axis while increases and decreases in $CMRO_2$ are indicated along the horizontal axis. A drug that has no effect on CBF or $CMRO_2$, such as sodium chloride, would occupy the intersection point. (From McKay RD: Head Trauma. In Newfield P, Cottrell J [eds]: *Neuroanesthesia: Clinical and Physiological Essentials.* Boston: Little, Brown, 1983. P 318.)

27
Syncope

DEFINITION

Syncope is defined as the sudden, reversible loss of consciousness (LOC), usually accompanied by generalized muscle weakness. In contrast, faintness refers to the sensation of impending LOC. Other conditions confused with syncope include cerebrovascular disturbances, hypoglycemia, seizures, and hyperventilation syndrome.

Syncope occurs when cerebral blood flow is reduced, leading to impairment of cerebral metabolism. Therefore, factors that decrease the quantity of blood to the brain produce syncope. These factors include decreased ventricular preload, inadequate vasoconstrictor mechanisms, reduced cardiac output, and cardiac arrhythmias.

ETIOLOGY
I. Decreased ventricular preload (see Chap. 13)
   A. Hypovolemia (acute hemorrhage, dehydration, diuresis, third-space losses)
   B. Decreased venous return
      1. Patient position (sitting, reverse Trendelenburg)
      2. Regional anesthesia (subarachnoid or epidural blockade)
      3. Atrial myxoma
      4. Drugs (direct vasodilators, alpha-adrenergic blockade)
      5. Decreased right ventricular (RV) output (pulmonary embolism, pulmonary hypertension)
      6. Cardiac tamponade

II. Inadequate vasoconstrictor mechanisms
   A. Vasodepressor (vasovagal)
   B. Autonomic insufficiency (Shy-Drager syndrome, dysautonomias, diabetic autonomic neuropathy)
   C. Sympathectomy (surgical, antihypertensive medication)
   D. Carotid sinus syncope
III. Reduced cardiac output
   A. Decreased left ventricular (LV) output (aortic stenosis [AS], idiopathic hypertrophic subaortic stenosis [IHSS], myocardial infarction)
   B. Drugs (beta-adrenergic blockers, calcium entry blockers)
IV. Cardiac arrhythmias
   A. Bradyarrhythmias
   B. Tachyarrhythmias
   C. Heart block (second degree, third degree [complete heart block])
   D. Prolonged Q–T interval (congenital, drug-induced [procainamide, quinidine])

DISCUSSION

Thorough history and physical examination are the initial steps in diagnosis. The effect of posture is a cardinal feature of syncope secondary to inadequate vasoconstrictor mechanisms. It may be familial (dysautonomias), idiopathic (Shy-Drager syndrome), or related to other disease states (alcoholic or diabetic autonomic neuropathy). Syncope that occurs in the recumbent position is invariably due to transient complete heart block (also called Stokes-Adams attacks); in all other cases of syncope, the patient is either sitting or standing. Patients with AS or IHSS develop exertional syncope, since cardiac output is fixed in the face of peripheral vasodilation. Patients with congenital nerve deafness may have a prolonged Q–T interval, leading to ventricular tachyarrhythmias.

Women with menometrorrhagia may be hypovolemic due to excessive blood loss. Syncope related to Valsalva maneuvers, such as coughing or urination, is occasionally seen in the elderly. Syncope due to carotid sinus sensitivity may be triggered by a tight-fitting collar, by turning the head to one side, or by shaving the area over the affected carotid sinus.

Drugs may lead to syncope through a variety of different mechanisms. The drug most noted to cause excessive postural hypotension and syncope is prazosin. It occurs 30 to 90 minutes following the first dose of the drug, particularly when the dose is 2 mg or greater. Other antihypertensive medications, such as hydralazine or methyldopa, interfere with vasoconstrictor mechanisms, producing a chemical sympathectomy. Beta-adrenergic blockers (especially propranolol), and calcium-entry blockers (notably verapamil) can reduce cardiac output. Nitrates and the residual effects of local anesthetics from regional blockade cause vasodilation, leading to decreased venous return. Diuretics, particularly potent agents such as furosemide, can produce hypovolemia. Antiarrhythmic medications (quinidine, procainamide) can prolong the Q–T interval, predisposing the patient to ventricular tachycardia (torsades de pointes).

Physical findings are of the utmost importance in diagnosis. Heart rate and blood pressure should be measured while the patient is both lying and standing. A drop in blood pressure (greater than 10 mm Hg) with an increase in heart rate (greater than 20 beats/minute) occurs when hypovolemia is present. If the blood pressure drops but the heart rate does not increase, autonomic dysfunction, secondary to either neuropathy or drugs, is likely. An extremely rapid (greater than 180 beats/minute) or slow (less than 50 beats/minute) heart rate may produce impairment of the cardiac output, leading to decreased cerebral perfusion. Auscultation of the heart may reveal a systolic ejection murmur consistent with AS or IHSS; a slowed carotid upstroke is indicative of significant AS.

Initial laboratory studies to order include hematocrit, glucose, and electrocardiogram (ECG). A patient may be anemic and hypovolemic from chronic blood loss. A low serum glucose can occur in diabetics or in patients with reactive hypoglycemia. The ECG may reveal an acute myocardial infarction, bradyarrhythmias, tachyarrhythmias, premature atrial or ventricular beats, or a prolonged Q–T interval; however, usually the ECG is normal. If an arrhythmia is suspected, 24-hour Holter monitoring can document transient arrhythmias or heart block. If poor LV function, valvular heart disease, IHSS, atrial myxoma, or pericardial effusion with tamponade is considered likely, an echocardiogram should be performed.

If all of these evaluations are negative, the most likely diagnosis is vasodepressor syncope, or the common faint. It often occurs in young females and frequently occurs during emotional stress, pain, or following a shocking accident. The patient quickly regains consciousness when placed in a supine position with the legs elevated.

SELECTED READING

Manolis AS, Linzer M, Salem D, Estes NA III: Syncope: Current diagnostic evaluation and management. *Ann Intern Med* 112 : 850, 1990.

IV
Gastrointestinal

28
Postoperative Jaundice

DEFINITION

Jaundice is characterized by hyperbilirubinemia with deposition of bile pigments in the skin, sclera, and mucous membranes; the resulting yellow appearance is also called icterus. The causes of jaundice can be divided into three categories: (1) prehepatic, due to excessive hemoglobin breakdown or impaired hepatic uptake of bilirubin, (2) intrahepatic, due to hepatocellular disease, and (3) posthepatic, due to obstruction of bilirubin excretion.

ETIOLOGY
  I. Prehepatic
     A. Intravascular hemolysis or trauma (transfusion reactions, autoimmune hemolysis, malfunctioning prosthetic heart valve, disseminated intravascular coagulation [DIC], glucose-6-phosphate dehydrogenase [G-6-PD] deficiency)
     B. Absorption of hematoma
     C. Bilirubin overload from stored blood
     D. Gilbert's syndrome
     E. Crigler-Najjar types I and II
     F. Neonatal jaundice
  II. Intrahepatic (hepatocellular)
     A. Viral hepatitis (hepatitis A, B, C, Epstein-Barr virus, cytomegalovirus)
     B. Drug toxicity (halothane, phenothiazines, methyldopa, estrogens, phenytoin, carbon tetrachloride)

   C. Hypoxemia
   D. Sepsis
   E. Preexisting liver disease/cirrhosis (alcoholic [Laennac's], Wilson's disease)
   F. Benign postoperative intrahepatic cholestasis
   G. Dubin-Johnson syndrome
   H. Rotor syndrome
   I. Intrahepatic cholestasis of pregnancy
   J. Decreased hepatic perfusion (shock, congestive heart failure [CHF], intraoperative hypotension, upper abdominal surgery)
III. Posthepatic (obstructive): obstruction of the common bile duct (tumor, stricture, stone, pancreatitis)

DISCUSSION

Most bilirubin is a byproduct of hemoglobin catabolism. The initial steps produce unconjugated (or indirect) bilirubin, a form that is lipid-soluble and therefore cannot be excreted by the kidneys. Normally, unconjugated bilirubin is the predominant type in the blood. The next steps include hepatic uptake by the enzyme glucuronyl transferase, conjugation with glucuronide to a water-soluble form called conjugated (or direct) bilirubin, and excretion via the common bile duct. The total bilirubin is a combination of conjugated and unconjugated bilirubin; for jaundice to become clinically evident, the total bilirubin usually exceeds 2.0 to 2.5 mg/dl.

Therefore, when a patient is jaundiced, the first step in evaluation is to compare the relative amounts of unconjugated and conjugated bilirubin. Prehepatic causes produce an unconjugated hyperbilirubinemia, while posthepatic problems produce a conjugated hyperbilirubinemia. Intrahepatic disorders lead to a mixed picture. Serial measurements of serum glutamic-oxaloacetic and glutamic-pyruvic transaminases (SGOT and SGPT) and alkaline phosphatase will further distinguish the specific category of hepatic dysfunction (Table 28-1). Another

Table 28-1. Hepatobiliary Disorders Classification
Based on Liver Function Tests

Dysfunction	Bilirubin	Transaminases	Alkaline Phosphatase
Prehepatic	Unconjugated	Normal	Normal
Intrahepatic	Conjugated > unconjugated	Elevated	Normal to Slightly ↑
Posthepatic	Conjugated	Normal to slightly ↑	Elevated

clue is whether bilirubin is detected in the urine; its presence suggests a conjugated hyperbilirubinemia.

In the first category, prehepatic jaundice, the unconjugated bilirubin level is elevated secondary to either excessive breakdown of hemoglobin or impaired hepatic uptake of bilirubin. Overload of hemoglobin byproducts occurs with (1) intravascular hemolysis or trauma (major transfusion reaction, DIC, G-6-PD deficiency), (2) absorption of large hematomas, or (3) massive transfusion of stored blood. Laboratory findings of intravascular hemolysis include anemia, low serum haptoglobin, hemoglobinemia, and hemoglobinuria; the last causes urine to turn pink. G-6-PD deficiency is seen in patients of Mediterranean descent when exposed to oxidizing agents, such as chloroquine or methylene blue. In cases of DIC, the prothrombin time, partial thromboplastin time, and fibrin degregation products are elevated while the plalelet count is depressed. With transfusions, it should be noted that 1 unit of fresh whole blood contains approximately 250 mg of bilirubin, an amount that increases as the age of the unit increases. It is the most likely cause of jaundice immediately following massive transfusion.

Several acquired or genetic abnormalities of the enzyme glucuronyl transferase can lead to jaundice. Low activity levels produce neonatal jaundice, which presents between the second and fifth days of life; the enzyme activity is further inhibited by hormones found in breast milk. This condition resolves with normal maturation of the liver or with cessation of breast feeding. Gilbert's syndrome (mild decreases in levels of glucuronyl transferase) and Crigler-Najjar types I and II (severe and moderate deficiencies, respectively) are genetic disorders. Gilbert's syndrome is usually asymptomatic and is often discovered on routine biochemical screens. In contrast, Crigler-Najjar type I leads to death in the first year of life, while type II is intermediate in severity.

Posthepatic, or obstructive, jaundice produces marked elevations in conjugated bilirubin and alkaline phosphatase. It is almost always due to obstruction of the common bile duct secondary to tumors, strictures, or stones.

The third category is intrahepatic, or hepatocellular, jaundice. Hepatocellular disease causes interference with all three steps of bilirubin metabolism (hepatic uptake, conjugation, and excretion). However, since excretion is the rate-limiting step and usually is impaired the most, conjugated hyperbilirubinemia predominates. In addition, SGOT and SGPT are elevated.

Initial evaluation of the jaundiced patient with intrahepatic dysfunction includes a thorough review of the past medical history for evidence of alcohol abuse (cirrhosis, alcoholic hepatitis), intravenous drug abuse (viral hepatitis), previous blood transfusions (viral hepatitis), exposure to drugs or toxins known to produce hepatitis (methyldopa, carbon tetrachloride), or recent pregnancy. It is estimated that up to 7 percent of patients who receive blood or blood products may develop hepatic dysfunction. Serologic studies can detect acute or chronic infections by hepatitis A, B, or C, cytomegalovirus, or Epstein-Barr virus. Hereditary conditions, such as Dubin-Johnson and Rotor's syndromes, may result in intrahepatic jaundice. Both conditions, transmitted as autosomal traits, have an excellent prognosis.

In addition, the patient's medical record should be reviewed for evidence of sepsis, profound hypotension, hypoxemia, shock, or congestive heart failure. A condition referred to as benign postoperative intrahepatic cholestasis has been described in the elderly after extensive surgery, particularly when complicated by hypotension, hypoxemia, or massive blood transfusions. It usually appears 1 to 14 days postoperatively and may persist for 2 to 4 weeks. Other liver function tests may be minimally impaired.

Finally, a condition termed halothane hepatitis is characterized by elevated liver function tests, fever, eosinophilia, and rarely, massive hepatic necrosis; severe liver damage is estimated to occur in 1 of every 22,000 to 35,000 cases after halothane administration. It appears most commonly in middle-aged, obese females who receive repeated exposure to halothane while it is exceedingly rare in children. Although the exact mechanism of injury is unclear, the leading theory is that it is due to an autoimmune reaction. It should be considered a diagnosis of exclusion, as it develops considerably less frequently than unsuspected liver disease in asymptomatic adults. In a 1-year study of elective surgical admissions, preoperative serum transaminase levels were determined. The incidence of elevated enzymes was approximately 1 : 700, with the incidence of overt jaundice about 1 : 2540. Therefore, preoperative liver dysfunction is fairly frequent, which makes postoperative diagnosis more difficult, since liver function tests are rarely obtained on elective surgical patients preoperatively.

SELECTED READING

Evans C, Evans M, Pollack AV: The incidence and causes of postoperative jaundice: A prospective study. *Br J Anaesth* 46 : 520, 1974.

Kartsonis A, Reddy KR, Manten HD, et al: Postoperative jaundice as a clue to unrecognized biliary tract obstruction. *J Clin Gastroenterol* 9 : 666, 1987.

Schiff L: Jaundice: Clinical pearls and perils revisited. *J Clin Gastroenterol* 9 : 383, 1987.

29
Nausea and Vomiting

DEFINITION

Nausea and vomiting, two of the most common conditions seen by anesthesia personnel, are so closely related that they are often considered together. Nausea is the feeling of the imminent desire to vomit, while vomiting is the forceful expulsion of gastric contents. Vomiting should be distinguished from regurgitation, the passive expulsion of food without nausea. Regurgitation is due to esophageal stricture or lower esophageal sphincter incompetence.

The etiologies of nausea and vomiting are extremely diverse, and classification is difficult, since the mechanisms leading to these symptoms are poorly understood in many disorders. However, the causes can be categorized according to the organ system triggering nausea and vomiting; they are (1) neurologic/psychogenic, (2) metabolic/endocrine, and (3) gastrointestinal/hepatic.

ETIOLOGY
I. Neurologic/psychogenic
   A. Increased intracranial pressure
   B. Drugs (apomorphine, narcotics, anesthetic agents)
   C. Emotional stress (anxiety, depression)
   D. Pain (surgical, myocardial infarction, renal colic)
   E. Acute febrile illness
   F. Drug toxicity (digoxin, theophylline)
   G. Neurologic disorders (migraine headaches,
      Ménière's disease)
   H. Hypotension

II. Metabolic/endocrine
   A. Electrolyte abnormalities (hyponatremia, hypercalcemia)
   B. Uremia
   C. Pregnancy
   D. Diabetic ketoacidosis
   E. Adrenal insufficiency
   F. Hypothyroidism
III. Gastrointestinal/hepatic
   A. Gastroenteritis (viral, food poisoning)
   B. Drugs (aspirin, codeine, erythromycin)
   C. Gastrointestinal pathology (appendicitis, cholecystitis, peptic ulcers)
   D. Hepatic failure
   E. Acute hepatitis

DISCUSSION

Nausea and vomiting are nonspecific symptoms, and since the causes are diverse, it is impossible to follow a specific diagnostic plan. However, many causes can be eliminated by carefully reviewing the history and medication record. Nausea and vomiting are often associated with surgical gastrointestinal pathology, such as cholecystitis and appendicitis, and nonsurgical diseases, including viral gastroenteritis, food poisoning, and acute hepatitis. Other historical findings of importance are hepatic failure, renal failure, and adrenal or thyroid disease. Central nervous system lesions that produce nausea and vomiting usually occur with other symptoms such as lethargy (increased intracranial pressure), headache (migraines), and vertigo (labyrinthine disease). Patients in diabetic ketoacidosis often present with acute abdominal pain, nausea, and vomiting; it is frequently the initial presentation of diabetes mellitus in children. Pain, anxiety, acute febrile illness, and hypotension secondary to regional anesthesia (subarachnoid or epidural anesthesia) can also lead to nausea and vomiting.

Drugs may produce nausea and vomiting through various mechanisms. Aspirin and codeine cause direct irritation to the gastric mucosa. Routine doses of narcotics stimulate the chemotactic trigger zone in the medulla, resulting in nausea and vomiting. Digoxin and theophylline produce nausea and vomiting at toxic levels; if nausea and vomiting occur in patients on either of these medications, serum drug levels should be measured. In the postoperative period, anesthetic agents such as volatile gases and nitrous oxide are common causes of nausea and vomiting, particularly when used in conjunction with narcotics.

Laboratory studies may help reveal correctable causes of nausea and vomiting. Hyponatremia and hypercalcemia may lead to nausea and vomiting; both electrolyte derangements may worsen from vomiting and additional fluid and electrolyte losses. Hyponatremia may develop following transurethral resection of the prostate. A pregnancy test may be indicated in women of childbearing age who present with nausea and vomiting. Other tests that may be beneficial in diagnosis include electrocardiogram (myocardial ischemia/ infarction), renal and hepatic function tests, and arterial blood gases (if an acid-base disturbance, such as diabetic ketoacidosis, is suspected).

Certain factors predispose to postoperative nausea and vomiting. They include (1) age (highest incidence in children and adolescents), (2) sex (females two to four times greater than males), (3) obesity, (4) previous history of postoperative nausea and vomiting, (5) premedication (greater with narcotics), (6) duration of anesthesia (the longer the procedure, the greater the incidence), and (7) site of operation (greatest in ophthalmologic, middle ear, and gynecologic surgery).

SELECTED READING

Forrest JB, Beattie WS, Goldsmith CH: Risk factors for nausea and vomiting after general anaesthesia. *Can J Anaesth* 37 : S90, 1990.
Palazzo MGA, Strunin L: Anaesthesia and emesis: I. Etiology. *Can Anaesth Soc J* 31 : 178, 1984.

V
Renal

30
Oliguria/Anuria

DEFINITION

In normal, awake individuals, oliguria is defined as urine output less than 400 ml/24 hours or less than 0.5 ml/kg/hour. The volume of urine considered oliguria in an anesthesized patient is not known, although the above amounts are usually applied. The etiology of oliguria can be divided into prerenal, renal, or postrenal causes. Anuria is the total absence of urine output; it results almost exclusively from postrenal causes.

ETIOLOGY
  I. Prerenal (inadequate renal perfusion)
     A. Hypovolemia (dehydration, hemorrhage, third-space losses)
     B. Decreased cardiac output
     C. Mechanical impairment of renal blood flow (aortic cross clamp)
     D. Hypotension (sepsis, anaphylaxis)
 II. Renal
     A. Renal failure (acute or chronic)
     B. Syndrome of inappropriate antidiuretic hormone (SIADH) secretion
     C. Hemolytic transfusion reaction
     D. Release of myoglobin (crush injury, malignant hyperthermia)
     E. Hepatorenal syndrome
III. Postrenal
     A. Obstruction of urinary catheter
     B. Benign prostatic hypertrophy

C. Impaired bladder drainage (Trendelenburg's position)
D. Extravasation due to bladder rupture
E. Bilateral ureteral obstruction
F. Epidural narcotics

DISCUSSION

The first step in evaluating oliguria is to ensure the patency of the lower urinary tract. Anuria almost always results from catheter obstruction or impaired bladder drainage due to patient position. The catheter should be flushed, and if uncertainty exists, should be replaced. Bladder rupture should be suspected if the patient was involved in an automobile accident while wearing a seat belt or if instrumentation of the bladder has occurred recently. Anuria following regional anesthesia with local anesthetics or narcotics may be due to delayed recovery of autonomic function to the bladder. Acute urinary retention in these circumstances may be more common in elderly males who have benign prostatic hypertrophy, although it can occur in normal individuals.

The cause of oliguria in the operating room is often readily apparent from history (chronic renal failure) or specific events (aortic cross clamping, blood transfusion). Myoglobinuria should be suspected in patients who have had crush injuries with massive tissue damage. In these individuals the urine will be pink and myoglobin will be identified on laboratory study of a urine sample. The hepatorenal syndrome is discussed in Chapter 32.

More commonly, however, the problem lies in determining whether oliguria is due to hypovolemia, decreased cardiac output, or SIADH. SIADH is characterized by hyponatremia, fluid retention, and oliguria. It is "inappropriate" because urine osmolality is greater than plasma osmolality. Multiple conditions can cause SIADH, including malignant and nonmalignant pulmonary diseases, central nervous system disorders, and drugs (morphine, oxytocin) (see Table 39-1). In patients under general anesthesia, SIADH is often due to pain, drugs, or positive-pressure ventilation. It should be emphasized that SIADH is a diagnosis of exclusion.

Next, one should determine whether oliguria is due to hypovolemia or decreased cardiac output. Aggressive treatment is important for patients who are at high risk for developing acute renal failure. High-risk patients include the elderly, those with coexisting renal or hepatic disease, and patients undergoing high-risk procedures such as cardiac or major vascular surgery. Healthy young patients who are not at risk for acute renal failure and who develop transient oliguria need only to be observed.

Initially, patients should receive a fluid volume challenge with 500 ml of a balanced salt solution. A brisk diuresis suggests hypovolemia as the cause of oliguria. If diuresis does not occur and if the patient is at risk for developing congestive heart failure, monitoring the cardiac filling pressures with a pulmonary artery catheter should be considered. If occlusion pressures are normal, further fluids can be given; if pressures are elevated and cardiac output is low, inotropic support (dopamine) may be needed. Diuretics (e.g., furosemide) should not be administered for oliguria unless hypovolemia has been ruled out.

SELECTED READING

Tonnesen A: Diagnosis and management of perioperative oliguria. *ASA Refresher Courses Anesthesiol* 18 : 299, 1990.

Tilney NL, Lazarus JM: Acute renal failure in surgical patients: Causes, clinical patterns, and care. *Surg Clin North Am* 63 : 357, 1983.

31
Polyuria

DEFINITION

Polyuria is defined in an adult as a urine volume greater than 3 liters/day. Causes of polyuria arise from three general problems: (1) fluid overload, (2) defect in renal water handling or (3) defect in secretion of antidiuretic hormone (ADH) (central or neurogenic diabetes insipidus [DI]).

ETIOLOGY

I. Fluid overload
   A. Intravenous fluids
   B. Primary polydipsia (compulsive water drinking)
II. Defect in renal water handling
   A. Osmotic diuresis (mannitol, glucose, angiographic contrast media)
   B. Diuretics (furosemide)
   C. Diuretic phase of acute tubular necrosis
   D. Postobstructive diuresis
   E. Nephrogenic diabetes insipidus
      1. Tubulointerstitial disease (pyelonephritis, analgesic abuse, sickle cell, sarcoidosis)
      2. Drugs or toxins (lithium, amphotericin B, phenytoin, propoxyphene, fluoride toxicity, demeclocycline)
      3. Electrolyte disturbances (hypokalemia, hypercalcemia)
III. Defects in secretion of antidiuretic hormone
   A. Craniofacial trauma
   B. Brain tumor

C. Central nervous system infection
D. Inflammation (sarcoidosis)
E. Vascular disorder (postpartum pituitary necrosis)
F. Post—neurosurgical procedure

DISCUSSION

The major causes of polyuria are fluid overload and defects in renal water handling. Fluid overload is most often due to aggressive administration of intravenous fluids; therefore, the medical record should be reviewed to calculate the amount of fluid given preoperatively. Primary polydipsia, which mimics neurogenic DI, is a diagnosis of exclusion. Defects in renal water handling are most commonly due to (1) osmotic diuresis from glucosuria (in poorly controlled diabetics), mannitol, and angiographic contrast dye, or (2) potent loop diuretics, such as furosemide. Other causes include post-obstructive diuresis and the recovery phase of acute tubular necrosis. Although the exact mechanism leading to post-obstructive uropathy is unclear, the resulting diuresis can produce marked fluid and electrolyte losses. The remaining categories are nephrogenic and neurogenic DI. Nephrogenic DI occurs when the kidneys fail to respond to normal or elevated levels of ADH. In contrast, with neurogenic DI, the kidney's response to ADH is normal, but the intrinsic level of ADH is low. In both cases, the urine osmolality is low, ranging from 50 to 200 mOsm/liter.

In most cases, the diagnosis can be established by a thorough preoperative history and review of the medical record. Nephrogenic DI usually results from a variety of drugs, toxins, or tubulointerstitial diseases. Electrolyte disturbances can produce a reversible form of nephrogenic DI. The major culprits are chronic hypokalemia and acute hypercalcemia. In these cases, the renal disorder develops slowly over the course of days or weeks, and polyuria is present preoperatively. Neurogenic DI develops after a significant central nervous system insult, such as trauma, tumor, infection, or inflammation. An idiopathic form of neurogenic DI occurs sporadically and usually presents in childhood.

The most difficult diagnostic situation occurs when a trauma patient with head injury develops polyuria in the operating room. Quite often, the patient has received mannitol and furosemide for treatment of cerebral edema and large quantities of crystalloid for resuscitation. If the serum sodium is high (greater than 150 mEq/liter), the problem is likely neurogenic DI; often, however, the sodium level is within the normal range. If the urine osmolality is inappropriately low compared to serum osmolality, neurogenic DI is likely. Measuring urine electrolytes is usually not helpful, particularly if the patient has received any diuretics. Polyuria secondary to mannitol and furosemide would be likely if diuresis was temporally related to drug administration. Fluid overload may be diagnosed by monitoring central venous or pulmonary artery pressures. If the diagnosis is still uncertain or if neurogenic DI is suspected, aqueous vasopressin can be given either intramuscularly or intravenously.

SELECTED READING

Baden JM, Mazze RI: Polyuria. In *Complications in Anesthesiology*. Philadelphia: Lippincott, 1983. Pp 415–422.

Baylis PH, Gill GV: The investigation of polyuria. *Clin Endocrinol Metab* 13 : 295, 1984.

32
Azotemia

DEFINITION

Blood urea nitrogen (BUN) is a byproduct of protein catabolism. It is almost exclusively eliminated by the kidneys via glomerular filtration, with some back diffusion from the tubular lumen to the peritubular blood. Normal values for BUN are 10 to 20 mg/dl. Azotemia (*azo*, "containing nitrogen") is defined as an elevation in blood urea nitrogen, while uremia implies an increase in products of protein breakdown associated with specific signs and symptoms of renal failure (fluid overload, electrolyte imbalance, anemia, retention of toxins). Azotemia is due to either increased protein metabolism or decreased urea clearance; it can be divided into prerenal, renal, or postrenal causes.

ETIOLOGY

I. Prerenal
   A. Decreased cardiac output (myocardial infarction, congestive heart failure, pericardial tamponade)
   B. Hypovolemia (hemorrhagic, diuretics, severe dehydration, third-space losses)
   C. Hypotension (sepsis, hypovolemia)
   D. Catabolic states (burns, steroid administration)
   E. Gastrointestinal bleeding
   F. High dietary protein (total parenteral nutrition [TPN], high-protein tube feedings)
II. Renal (uremia)
   A. Acute renal failure (acute tubular necrosis, acute glomerulonephritis)

B. End-stage renal disease
C. Hepatorenal syndrome
III. Postrenal
   A. Prostatic obstruction
   B. Bilateral ureteral obstruction (tumor, valves)

DISCUSSION

Thorough history and physical examination will reveal many of the causes of azotemia. The diagnosis of end-stage renal disease is usually apparent. Preoperative causes of prerenal azotemia include catabolic states (burns, steroid administration), increased protein intake (TPN, tube feedings), and gastrointestinal bleeding. Gastrointestinal bleeding that leads to azotemia usually originates in the upper gastrointestinal tract; azotemia is due to a combination of increased protein load plus decreased intravascular volume. If azotemia is due to postrenal obstruction, it is almost always accompanied by anuria. Placement of a Foley catheter will relieve obstruction secondary to benign prostatic hypertrophy, the most common cause of postrenal azotemia. Ultrasound studies can help diagnose bilateral ureteral obstruction with concomitant hydronephrosis.

If the above are negative, prerenal azotemia must be distinguished from acute renal failure. The first step in diagnosis is to obtain BUN and serum creatinine levels. A BUN-to-creatinine ratio greater than 10 suggests a prerenal cause, while a ratio less than 10 suggests a renal disorder. The creatinine clearance can be estimated using the following equation:

$$C_{cr} \text{ (ml/min)} = \frac{0.7 \; (U_{cr} \text{ mg/dl}) \; (\text{vol liters/day})}{P_{cr} \text{ mg/dl}}$$

Where C_{cr} = creatinine clearance
U_{cr} = urine creatinine
vol = volume of urine
P_{cr} = plasma creatinine

Calculating the creatinine clearance is useful in patients with stable serum creatinine levels. The normal creatinine clearance is 75 to 80 ml/minute. Moderate renal impairment reduces creatinine clearance to 35 to 40 ml/minute; when the clearance is less than 5 ml/minute, dialysis is indicated. However, calculations are not valid in acute renal failure, where the serum creatinine is rapidly changing.

Next, urine electrolytes should be measured. A urine sodium less than 20 mEq/liter indicates prerenal azotemia, as the kidney avidly resorbs sodium to maintain intravascular volume. A urine sodium greater than 40 mEq/liter suggests acute tubular necrosis, as the damaged tubules are unable to resorb sodium. Other urine indices that help distinguish prerenal azotemia from acute renal failure are listed in Table 32-1. It should be noted that urine electrolytes and osmolality are not valid when the patient has received diuretics, such as furosemide, as these drugs produce an elevated urine sodium when tubules are normal.

Two other calculations that can help distinguish prerenal from renal azotemia are the renal failure index and the fractional excretion of sodium (Table 32-1). Both are more sensitive than the urine sodium alone. However, since these calculations are based on urine sodium levels, the results are not accurate following diuretic administration.

One condition that mimics prerenal azotemia is the hepatorenal syndrome. In this syndrome, patients with severe hepatic cirrhosis develop progressive azotemia and oliguria with a urine sodium less than 10. It usually follows a large and rapid change in intravascular volume, such as that caused by hemorrhage, vigorous diuresis, or paracentesis. Renal dysfunction develops in the absence of clinical, laboratory, or anatomic evidence of other causes of renal failure. It appears that altered renal hemodynamics are responsible for this disorder. Attempts at intravascular volume expansion can be tried, although this rarely is successful. Once this syndrome develops, death usually ensues.

Treatment should be directed at the causes of prerenal azotemia. It should be approached aggressively, as many of

Table 32-1. Urine Findings in Prerenal Azotemia and Acute Renal Failure

Laboratory Test	Prerenal Azotemia	Acute Renal Failure
Urine osmolality (mOsm/kg)	> 500	< 400
Urine sodium (mEq/liter)	< 20	> 40
Urine/plasma creatinine	> 40	< 20
Renal failure index[†]	< 1	> 2
Fractional excretion[‡] of filtered sodium	< 1	2
Urine sediment	Normal or occasional granular casts	Brown granular casts, cellular debris

[†] $\dfrac{Urine\ Na\ (mEq/liter)}{Urine/plasma\ creatinine}$.

[‡] $\dfrac{Urine\ Na/serum\ Na}{Urine\ creatinine/serum\ creatinine}$.

Source: Anderson RJ, Schrier RW: Acute renal failure. In Petersdorf RG, Adams RD, Braunwald E, et al: *Harrison's Principles of Internal Medicine*, 10th ed. New York: McGraw-Hill, 1983. P 1606.

the causes of prerenal azotemia, such as hypovolemia or decreased cardiac output, will lead to acute renal failure secondary to acute tubular necrosis if left untreated. This transition to renal failure is more likely when other insults, such as angiographic dye, aminoglycosides, or aortic cross clamping, are superimposed on prerenal azotemia.

Intravascular volume should be optimized to maintain renal perfusion with either crystalloid or colloid solutions. Placement of a pulmonary artery catheter may be necessary if aggressive treatment with fluids would be detrimental, if decreased cardiac output is felt to be a contributing factor, or if hemodynamics are unstable. Once the volume status has been optimized, dopamine may be added. Dopamine may be helpful in two ways: (1) by enhancing cardiac output through inotropic effects and (2) by helping to improve renal perfusion via dopaminergic receptors in the kidney.

SELECTED READING

Myers BD, Moran SM: Hemodynamically mediated acute renal failure. *N Engl J Med* 314 : 97, 1986.

Oken DE: On the differential diagnosis of acute renal failure. *Am J Med* 71 : 916, 1981.

Wilkes BM, Mailloux LU: Acute renal failure: Pathogenesis and prevention. *Am J Med* 80 : 1129, 1986.

33
Dark Urine

DEFINITION

Normally, urine is clear to golden yellow in color, depending on the amount of urobilinogen present. Any other color is abnormal and should be investigated. The appearance of the specimen can be divided according to color: red/pink, brown/blue, and dark orange.

ETIOLOGY

I. Red/pink
  A. Hematuria (tumor, trauma, glomerulonephritis)
  B. Hemoglobinuria (intravascular hemolysis)
  C. Myoglobinuria
  D. Drugs (phenolphthalein)
II. Brown/blue
  A. Porphyrias (acute intermittent porphyria)
  B. Alkaptonuria
  C. Drugs (methylene blue, indigo carmen)
III. Dark orange
  A. Bilirubin
  B. Concentrated urine (urobilinogen)
  C. Drugs (phenazopyridine, rifampin)

DISCUSSION

After color determination, the next step in diagnosis is to review the patient's history and medication record. Commonly used drugs that alter the color of urine include phenazopyridine, phenolphthalein (found in laxatives), and rifampin. Methylene blue or indigo carmen may have been given to the patient in the operating suite, especially during urologic or gynecologic procedures.

The history may indicate porphyrias (particularly acute intermittent porphyria [AIP]) or alkaptonuria as the underlying problem. AIP is an autosomal dominant disorder, due to partial deficiency of the enzyme uroporphyrinogen I synthase. It is characterized by acute attacks of abdominal pain or neuropsychiatric disturbances. These patients may present for emergency surgery with acute abdominal pain of unknown etiology. In addition, they may receive sodium pentothal for induction of general anesthesia; barbiturates are among the compounds that commonly precipitate AIP. The only clue to the diagnosis may be a change in urine color, from clear to dark brown, with standing. Other conditions that can trigger AIP include corticosteroids, excessive alcohol intake, and prolonged fasting (hypoglycemia).

Alkaptonuria is a rare disorder of tyrosine metabolism. It usually presents as degenerative arthritis during middle age. In the operating room, it may become evident when the urine darkens to brown with standing.

Blood, hemoglobin, or myoglobin will change the urine color to pink or red. Hematuria may be secondary to glomerular disease, tumor, trauma, or most commonly, manipulation of the urinary tract with an indwelling catheter or other instruments. Hemoglobinuria occurs after massive intravascular hemolysis overwhelms the haptoglobin scavenging system. Hemolysis may develop in patients with malfunctioning prosthetic heart valves, with autoantibodies antibodies to red blood cells, or with a major blood transfusion reaction. Myoglobinuria may develop following massive crush injuries or an episode of malignant hyperthermia.

The most common causes of dark orange urine, dehydration and contracted intravascular volume, are associated with oliguria and concentration of urobilinogen. When bile pigments produce the orange color, the underlying pathology is (1) posthepatic obstruction, secondary to tumors or common bile duct stones or (2) the obstructive phase of acute hepatitis.

SELECTED READING

Werman HA: The porphyrias. *Emerg Med Clin North Am* 7 : 927, 1989.

VI
Metabolic/Endocrine

34
Hyperthermia

DEFINITION

Hyperthermia is defined as an elevation in the body's core temperature to greater than 38.5°C. Hyperthermia leads to increased oxygen demand of tissues, with a concomitant rise in respiratory and cardiac work. Causes of hyperthermia can be divided into three major categories: (1) increased heat production, (2) decreased heat elimination, and (3) active warming.

ETIOLOGY

I. Increased heat production
   A. Infectious process (bacteremia, viremia)
   B. Metabolic disorders (malignant hyperthermia, thyrotoxicosis)
   C. Chemical reactions (polymerization of bone cement)
II. Decreased heat elimination
   A. Decreased sweating (anticholinergic medication)
   B. Dehydration
   C. Patient's coverings (drapes, plastic covers)
III. Active warming
   A. Elevated room temperature
   B. Heated humidification of airway
   C. Warming fluids (intravenous, irrigation)
   D. Heat lamps

DISCUSSION

Hyperthermia occurs much less frequently than hypothermia in the operating room; however, when it does develop, the cause must be discovered to determine whether the patient has malignant hyperthermia. In most cases, the combination of actively warming the patient (fluids, humidified airway gases) and blocking heat elimination (covering with surgical drapes) leads to hyperthermia. It is especially true in infants who have a high surface-volume ratio; as a result, they are vulnerable to warming from external sources. Anticholinergic medication contributes to decreased heat elimination by preventing sweating.

Increased heat production is the third cause of hyperthermia. An elevated temperature due to sepsis is usually apparent preoperatively. Occasionally, heat produced by polymerization of methylmethacrylate can transiently increase the patient's body temperature.

The major concern is whether the patient has malignant hyperthermia. Malignant hyperthermia is a metabolic disorder involving aberrant calcium metabolism in skeletal muscle cells. This condition, a true pharmacogenetic disease, develops in susceptible patients exposed to anesthetic triggering agents (succinylcholine, halothane). The initial manifestation is an increase in end-tidal carbon dioxide tension, followed by sinus tachycardia and profound metabolic and respiratory acidoses; hyperthermia is a late finding. An increase in a patient's temperature without an elevation in arterial carbon dioxide tension is *not* malignant hyperthermia. It may be difficult to distinguish malignant hyperthermia from thyrotoxicosis, or "thyroid storm." Usually a patient with thyrotoxicosis has either a history of thyroid disease or the stigmata of hyperthyroidism (weight loss, goiter, exophthalmos).

SELECTED READING

Greenberg C: Diagnosis and treatment of hyperthermia in the postanesthesia care unit. *Anesthesiol Clin North Am* 8 : 377, 1990.

Rosenberg H: Malignant hyperthermia. *41st Annual Refresher Course Lectures and Clinical Update Program*. American Society of Anesthesiologists. Lecture 245, pp 1–6.

35
Hypothermia

DEFINITION

Hypothermia is defined as a core temperature less than 35°C. Both organ function and drug metabolism are affected by declines in body temperature. Causes of hypothermia fall into three categories: (1) increased heat losses, (2) decreased heat production, and (3) deliberate hypothermia.

ETIOLOGY

I. Increased heat losses
 A. Low ambient environmental temperature
 B. Cold fluids (intravenous, irrigation)
 C. Cold operating room table
 D. Ventilation with dry gases
 E. Blood transfusions
 F. Vasodilation (anesthetic agents, regional anesthesia, spinal cord lesion)
 G. Increased surface-volume ratio (neonates, cachectic patients)
 H. Increased exposed surfaces (intraabdominal surgery, burns)
II. Decreased heat production
 A. Decreased shivering (muscle relaxants, neonates)
 B. Decreased muscle mass (elderly, cachectic patients)
 C. Hypothyroidism
 D. Anesthetic agents
 E. Central nervous system (CNS) diseases

III. Deliberate
  A. Extracorporeal circulation
  B. Neurosurgical procedures (cerebral aneurysm clipping)

DISCUSSION

Temperature is measured at several different sites, each with advantages and disadvantages. Axillary or skin temperatures are easily recorded but highly inaccurate due to variations in ambient room temperature and cutaneous blood flow. Rectal temperatures vary with splanchnic perfusion and do not necessarily reflect core temperature. Both tympanic membrane and nasopharyngeal thermometers record the temperature of blood perfusing the brain; however, these probes can cause perforation or bleeding. Upper esophageal temperatures, as recorded with a combined esophageal stethoscope/thermometer, measure the temperature of the respiratory gases, not the patient. Probably the most accurate temperatures are those recorded in the lower esophagus, urinary bladder, and pulmonary artery (excluding cases of pericardial irrigation during cardiac operations). In most cases, the precise temperature is not as important as trending changes.

A number of patient-specific factors contribute to hypothermia in the operating room. The first is the patient's size. Neonates, who have a surface-volume ratio 2 to 3 times greater than an adult's, lose heat more readily to the environment. The second factor is the patient's age, at both ends of the spectrum. Infants under 3 months old do not shiver; additional heat is produced from brown fat by nonshivering thermogenesis. The elderly lose heat to the environment more rapidly due to reduced ability to thermoregulate and are slower to rewarm postoperatively because of less muscle mass to produce heat by shivering. The third factor is body habitus; like neonates, cachectic patients have an increased surface-volume ratio and, like the elderly, have decreased heat production mechanisms.

A number of factors specific to either the operating room or the anesthetic technique contribute to hypothermia. First, it should be noted that heat loss occurs by four mechanisms: (1) radiation—loss of heat in the form of electromagnetic energy to colder objects, (2) convection—heat loss due to air currents, (3) conduction—heat loss to surfaces directly touching the body, and (4) evaporative—heat loss due to heat of vaporization.

The majority of heat loss comes from radiation to colder objects, such as the anesthesia machine. Rapid air turnover, as occurs in laminar airflow rooms, increases convective losses. Both can be reduced by warming the operating room and by covering the patient with blankets. Anesthetic agents increase radiant heat losses by producing vasodilation; this includes both general (isoflurane) and regional anesthesia (subarachnoid or epidural blocks). Similar to regional anesthesia, patients with high spinal cord lesions are poikilothermic. Evaporative heat loss from ventilating with dry gases accounts for up to 20 percent of the total heat loss. The heat of vaporization is 580 calories/g of water; since gases become fully saturated during respiration, a large amount of heat is expended to vaporize water. This loss can be attenuated by humidifying the gases or by adding an "artificial nose." Radiant and evaporative losses from exposed surfaces during intra-abdominal surgery or extensive skin grafting for burns contribute to hypothermia. Cold operating room tables increase conductive losses, which can be reduced by placing a warming blanket under the patient. These blankets are beneficial primarily in patients whose body surface area is less than 0.5 m^2 or who weigh less than 10 kg. In larger patients they contribute little to warming but may cause skin burns. Another cause of cooling, particularly in children, is using irrigation or intravenous fluids that are not warmed. When large quantities of blood are transfused, every effort should be made to warm them, since each unit is stored at 4°C.

Although hypothermia is mainly due to increased heat loss, a few factors contribute to decreased heat production.

Patients with hypothyroidism have a decreased basal metabolic rate. Certain CNS disorders and anesthetic agents can affect the hypothalamus, producing alterations in body temperature regulation. Muscle relaxants and regional anesthetics impair heat production by blocking shivering. The absence of shivering in patients with subarachnoid or epidural anesthesia prevents them from rewarming as fast as patients with the same core temperature who had general anesthesia. Deliberate hypothermia for cardiac or neurosurgical procedures is apparent.

Prevention of hypothermia is important for many reasons. First, low temperatures cause shivering, which increases oxygen consumption by up to 500 percent. Acidosis and hypoxia can develop, since increased oxygen demand coupled with elevated carbon dioxide production occurs in patients who may be unable to increase ventilation, due to either residual anesthetics or incisional pain. In addition, since the central hypothalamic shivering response is impaired below 32°C, patients rewarm more slowly. As the patient cools, the oxyhemoglobin dissociation curve shifts to the right, which decreases oxygen unloading to tissues. Secondly, at cold temperatures, drug metabolism is impaired and the CNS is sensitized to the effects of residual volatile and intravenous anesthetics, which delays awakening. Lastly, extremely low temperatures (less than 30°C) can lead to ventricular irritability and direct CNS depression. Below 28°C there is a significant risk of refractory ventricular fibrillation or asystole, the leading causes of death at cold temperatures.

SELECTED READING

Lilly RB Jr: Significance and recovery room management of post-anesthesia hypothermia and shivering. *Anesthesiol Clin North Am* 8 : 365, 1990.

Sladen R: Temperature regulation and anesthesia. *41st Annual Refresher Course Lectures and Clinical Update Program.* American Society of Anesthesiologists. Lecture 243, pp 1–7.

36
Metabolic Acidosis

DEFINITION

Metabolic acidosis is defined as a pH less than 7.35 in the absence of respiratory acidosis. It is caused by either an increase in nonvolatile acids or a loss of bicarbonate from the serum. The initial categorization is based on the presence or absence of an anion gap, which is calculated by the equation:

$$\text{Anion gap} = [Na^+] - [HCO_3^- + Cl^-]$$

Where $[Na^+]$ = sodium concentration
$[HCO_3^-]$ = bicarbonate concentration
$[Cl^-]$ = chloride concentration

The normal anion gap, 8 to 16 mEq/liter, is composed primarily of albumin, phosphates, and sulfates; an increase above this level represents unmeasured anions in the serum. The causes of metabolic acidosis can be divided into two categories: (1) increased and (2) normal anion gap.

ETIOLOGY

I. Increased anion gap
   A. Increased acid production
      1. Ketoacidosis (diabetic, alcoholic, starvation)
      2. Lactic acidosis
         a. Circulatory failure
         b. Respiratory failure

      c. Drugs (salicylates, paraldehyde, phenformin, cyanide)

      d. Other (liver failure, alcohol intake)

   3. Toxins (methanol, ethylene glycol)

  B. Renal failure—uremic acidosis

II. Normal anion gap (hyperchloremic)

  A. Renal tubular dysfunction

   1. Renal tubular acidosis (proximal, distal)

   2. Hypoaldosteronism

  B. Nonrenal disorders

   1. Diarrhea

   2. Ureterosigmoidostomy

   3. Carbonic anhydrase inhibitors (acetazolamide)

   4. Total parenteral nutrition (TPN)

   5. Increased acid intake (ammonium chloride)

DISCUSSION

Patients with metabolic acidosis have few symptoms that specifically indicate this disorder. If metabolic acidosis develops acutely, hyperventilation ensues to produce a compensatory respiratory alkalosis; this labored breathing pattern is referred to as Kussmaul's respirations. Acute acidosis may lead to confusion, stupor, or coma, along with decreased cardiac contractility and vasodilation. Arterial blood gases, serum electrolytes (primarily potassium, chloride, and bicarbonate), and serum glucose help establish the diagnosis.

The first grouping, increased anion gap acidosis, indicates that an acid with an anion other than chloride has accumulated. The chloride level remains normal while the bicarbonate level drops as hydrogen ions are buffered. Reviewing the history and medication record help distinguish whether the patient has ketoacidosis or lactic acidosis; if uncertain, serum ketones or lactate can be measured. Ketoacidosis develops when carbohydrate metabolism is impaired and fat metabolism increases. Diabetic ketoacidosis is often the initial manifestation of type I diabetes mellitus in children. It may also develop in diabetics when a concurrent illness, such as infection, renders them relatively insulin resistant. Starvation ketoacidosis is similar to, but usually less severe than diabetic ketoacidosis. Alcoholic ketoacidosis develops in heavy alcohol users who abruptly withdraw from alcohol and have inadequate caloric intake.

Lactic acidosis is the result of derangements in oxidative phosphorylation, due to tissue hypoxia or to uncoupling of phosphorylation from oxidation by drugs. The major cause is tissue hypoxia secondary to either decreased perfusion (circulatory failure) or hypoxemic hypoxia (respiratory failure). The decreased availability of oxygen causes cells to convert to anaerobic metabolism, with lactic acid accumulating as a byproduct.

Drugs can produce lactic acidosis. The classic example is phenformin, an oral hypoglycemic agent no longer available for clinical use. Salicylate intoxication produces respiratory alkalosis from direct stimulation of the ventilatory center, followed by metabolic acidosis caused by excessive lactate production. Paraldehyde, once used in the treatment of alcohol withdrawal, can produce metabolic acidosis when given in large quantities. Cyanide causes lactic acidosis secondary to impaired oxygen utilization at the cellular level. Cyanide is a byproduct of sodium nitroprusside metabolism and the combustion of synthetic compounds; it is a major contributor to metabolic acidosis following smoke inhalation.

Two toxins, ethylene glycol and methanol, are occasionally ingested by chronic alcoholics when ethanol is unavailable; both can produce an increased anion gap metabolic acidosis. Ethylene glycol, the main component of antifreeze, is metabolized to lactate, oxalate, and glycolate; central nervous system symptoms range from intoxication to convulsions and coma. Methanol is converted to formic acid and formaldehyde. Following methanol consumption, patients present acutely intoxicated with profound acidosis (secondary to formic acid) and impaired vision (secondary to formaldehyde). The presence of an osmolar gap (osmolar gap = measured − calculated osmolality) should heighten the suspicion that methanol has been ingested, since it produces metabolic acidosis with an elevated serum osmolality.

Renal failure is the second major cause of increased anion gap acidosis. Uremic acidosis is due to retention of phosphates, sulfates, and other solutes. Impairment of both hydrogen ion excretion and bicarbonate resorption contributes to the acidosis. In these patients, plasma bicarbonate levels range from 12 to 18 mmol/liter.

The second major category is normal anion gap acidosis; also referred to as hyperchloremic metabolic acidosis, it is caused by both renal and nonrenal disorders. With normal anion gap acidosis, there is either a failure to excrete acid (distal renal tubular acidosis [RTA]) or an excessive loss of bicarbonate (diarrhea, proximal renal tubular acidosis); these processes lead to renal conservation of chloride with subsequent hyperchloremia. Distal RTA occurs more frequently than proximal RTA; the latter occurs as part of Fanconi's syndrome. Diarrhea is by far the most frequent nonrenal cause in this grouping. Ureterosigmoidostomy produces metabolic acidosis by two mechanisms: (1) exchange of chloride for bicarbonate by intestinal epithelium and (2) development of renal disease, primarily pyelonephritis. Metabolic acidosis does not occur when ileal conduits are created.

Occasionally, drugs can cause a normal anion gap acidosis. Either excessive ammonium chloride ingestion or inadequate bicarbonate levels in TPN can produce it. Carbonic anhydrase inhibitors, such as acetazolamide, cause increased bicarbonate loss in the urine.

SUGGESTED READING

Brewer ED: Disorders of acid-base balance. *Pediatr Clin North Am* 37 : 429, 1990.

Kearns T, Wolfson AB: Metabolic acidosis. *Emerg Med Clin North Am* 7 : 823, 1989.

37
Metabolic Alkalosis

DEFINITION

Metabolic alkalosis is defined as a pH greater than 7.45; it develops secondary to an increase in the serum bicarbonate concentration. Bicarbonate arises from either the addition of base or the loss of acid. Causes of metabolic alkalosis fall into three general categories: (1) chloride-responsive due to intravascular volume depletion, (2) chloride-resistant primarily due to mineralocorticoid excess, and (3) increased alkali intake.

ETIOLOGY

  I. Chloride-responsive
     A. Gastrointestinal losses (vomiting, nasogastric suctioning)
     B. Diuretics (furosemide, thiazides)
     C. Posthypercapnic alkalosis
 II. Chloride-resistant
     A. Cushing's disease
     B. Hyperaldosteronism (primary, Bartter's syndrome)
     C. Adrenocorticotropic hormone (ACTH)–secreting tumors (bronchogenic carcinoma)
     D. Pseudohyperaldosteronism (Liddle's syndrome, licorice ingestion)
     E. Severe potassium depletion
III. Increased alkali intake
     A. Acute (bicarbonate administration, acetate in dialysis baths)
     B. Milk-alkali syndrome

DISCUSSION

Metabolic alkalosis is much less common than metabolic acidosis. In the majority of cases, the presence of alkalosis indicates that the patient either is volume depleted or has mineralocorticoid excess. It may be partly offset by a compensatory respiratory acidosis. However, this response is limited by hypoxia so the carbon dioxide level rarely rises above 50 to 55 mm Hg. Other disturbances caused by metabolic alkalosis include a decrease in the ionized calcium level and a shift of potassium into the intracellular pool.

Most cases of metabolic alkalosis are due to volume depletion. Vomiting and nasogastric suctioning produce alkalosis by two mechanisms. First, there is a loss of hydrochloric acid (HCl) from the stomach. As hydrogen ion (H^+) is lost, further hydrogen ions are generated by the parietal cells in the stomach; for each one hydrogen ion produced, one bicarbonate molecule enters the circulation. In addition, less chloride is available for reuptake by the kidney as a concomitant anion with sodium; subsequently, all the filtered bicarbonate is resorbed.

The second mechanism involves intravascular volume depletion. The decrease in intravascular volume triggers sodium resorption by the kidney. This process involves both the sodium-hydrogen and sodium-potassium exchange pumps. First, hydrogen ion is exchanged for sodium in the tubular lumen; the net effect is that almost all the filtered bicarbonate is resorbed. Second, volume contraction stimulates aldosterone release, which leads to sodium-potassium exchange and ultimately potassium depletion by the kidney. As potassium losses become severe, the exchange process shifts back in the direction of the sodium-hydrogen pump, which promotes further bicarbonate resorption. In addition, potassium depletion stimulates ammoniagenesis, resulting in the de novo synthesis of bicarbonate.

Diuretics produce metabolic alkalosis by both distal renal hydrogen ion losses and volume contraction. It may develop in patients treated with any diuretic except (1) acetazolamide, which specifically inhibits bicarbonate resorption, and (2) spironolactone and triamterene, which inhibit distal cation secretion.

Posthypercapnic alkalosis develops when patients with chronic respiratory acidosis have a rapid correction of the arterial carbon dioxide tension to normal. These patients had generated a compensatory metabolic alkalosis to help restore the pH to normal. Once the respiratory acidosis is cleared, the metabolic alkalosis remains; it takes several days for the elevated bicarbonate level to be excreted by the kidneys.

In patients with chloride-responsive metabolic alkalosis, the serum and urine chloride levels are low, with urine chloride less than 10 mEq/liter. The primary treatment consists of administering sodium chloride both to restore intravascular volume and to replenish serum chloride concentration. Once the chloride level is corrected, bicarbonate can be excreted by the kidney.

The second category, chloride-resistant metabolic alkalosis, is due to excessive mineralocorticoid activity. Alkalosis is generated by renal acid loss and maintained by potassium depletion; severe potassium depletion (serum levels less than 2 mEq/liter) may directly cause metabolic alkalosis. Alkalosis ranges from mild in patients with Cushing's disease or primary hyperaldosteronism to more severe in patients with marked hyperfunction secondary to ACTH-secreting tumors such as bronchogenic carcinoma. These patients are mildly volume expanded, and the urine chloride levels are greater than 20 mEq/liter. The condition is unresponsive to sodium chloride therapy; treatment consists of replacing potassium and correcting the underlying mineralocorticoid excess.

The third cause of metabolic alkalosis is excessive alkali administration, either intravenously (sodium bicarbonate) or orally (milk-alkali syndrome). Under these conditions, alkalosis cannot be maintained unless either renal function is impaired or large quantities of alkali are given.

SELECTED READING

Brewer ED: Disorders of acid-base balance. *Pediatr Clin North Am* 37 : 429, 1990.

Goodkin DA, Krishna GG, Narins RG: The role of anion gap in detecting and managing mixed acid-base disorders. *Clin Endocrinol Metab* 13 : 333, 1984.

38
Hypernatremia

DEFINITION

Hypernatremia is defined as a serum sodium concentration greater than 145 mEq/liter. Sodium, the major solute in the extracellular fluid (ECF), determines both ECF and plasma volume. When evaluating a patient with hypernatremia, one should determine whether the ECF volume is low, normal, or high. Causes of hypernatremia can be divided into three categories, based on the ECF volume: (1) hypovolemic, due to loss of hypotonic fluid, (2) isovolemic, due to loss of free water, and (3) hypervolemic, due to addition of sodium.

ETIOLOGY

I. Hypovolemic
   A. Renal
      1. Osmotic diuresis (glucose, mannitol, radiocontrast media)
      2. Diuretics (furosemide)
      3. Partial urinary tract obstruction
      4. Renal failure (acute, chronic)
   B. Miscellaneous
      1. Adrenal insufficiency (congenital, acquired)
      2. Gastrointestinal losses (gastroenteritis, diarrhea)
      3. Excessive sweating
      4. Respiratory losses (hyperventilation)
II. Isovolemic
   A. Neurogenic diabetes insipidus (DI) (idiopathic, neoplastic, infiltrative, trauma)

B. Nephrogenic diabetes insipidus (drugs, hypokalemia, hypercalcemia, sickle cell disease, sarcoidosis, pyelonephritis)

C. Mucocutaneous losses (fever, hypermetabolic states)

III. Hypervolemia

A. Sodium bicarbonate administration (cardiac arrest, lactic acidosis)

B. Sodium chloride injection (abortions)

C. Hypertonic infant formula

D. Dialysis baths

E. Mineralocorticoid excess (Cushing's disease, congenital adrenal hyperplasia)

DISCUSSION

The first step in diagnosis of hypernatremia is to determine the patient's volume status. Patients with hypovolemic hypernatremia have lost both water and sodium, with water losses exceeding solute losses. Signs of dehydration, such as decreased skin turgor, tachycardia, and orthostatic hypotension, are present. In contrast, patients with isovolemic hypernatremia have minimal signs of dehydration; since they have lost pure water without sodium, ECF is maintained near normal. Hypervolemic hypernatremia is the third possibility. These individuals have signs of volume overload, such as peripheral edema, since sodium and some water have been gained. In all three categories the ECF is hypertonic, which draws water out of cells. The major impact is on the central nervous system; intracellular dehydration leads to impaired mentation, lethargy, weakness, and coma. These patients may develop compulsive water drinking secondary to their hypertonic state.

The first category, hypovolemic hypernatremia, results from hypotonic fluid losses through the kidney, skin, respiratory, or gastrointestinal tract. Osmotic diuresis triggers renal losses, with the most common situations occurring (1) in diabetics with profound hyperglycemia and glucosuria and (2) in neurosurgical patients receiving mannitol for increased intracranial pressure. In diabetics, an elevated serum sodium concentration in the presence of hyperglycemia indicates that fluid losses have been substantial. Other renal causes include acute and chronic renal failure, partial urinary tract obstruction, and administration of potent diuretics, such as furosemide. Excessive sweating can occur in patients who vigorously exercise on hot days or in hot rooms. Sweat is hypotonic, containing one-third to one-fourth the sodium concentration of plasma. Diarrhea fluid, particularly in infants, is hypotonic; large losses can lead to hypovolemic hypernatremia. Lactulose therapy, used in the treatment of hepatic encephalopathy, produces a similar picture.

Most cases of isovolemic hypernatremia are secondary to problems with antidiuretic hormone (ADH). ADH is released from the posterior pituitary and acts on the kidney to increase free water resorption from the distal tubules and collecting ducts. Two abnormalities can occur: (1) the amount of hormone is decreased, producing neurogenic DI, or (2) the kidney is unresponsive to it, leading to nephrogenic DI. Neurogenic DI can occur with a variety of central nervous system disorders, such as head trauma, malignancy (primary or metastatic), cerebrovascular accidents, infiltrative processes, or infections. An idiopathic form develops either sporadically or is transmitted as an autosomal dominant trait. Nephrogenic DI results from a number of renal insults, including sickle cell disease, pyelonephritis, and sarcoidosis. Both hypercalcemia and hypokalemia render the kidney unresponsive to ADH. Overall, drugs are the most common cause of nephrogenic DI; they include lithium carbonate and demeclocycline, a tetracycline derivative. Fluoride nephrotoxicity secondary to methoxyflurane metabolism first presents as nephrogenic DI, which was the prime reason for its restriction from human use.

Other causes of isovolemic hypernatremia include excessive loss of fluid from the skin and respiratory tract. A common scenario is an elderly patient who suffers a stroke in the summer months; if living alone, this patient is unable to replace fluid losses adequately. Contributing to the problem is disturbed heat regulation, which is not uncommon following cerebrovascular accidents. Both febrile and hypermetabolic states have substantial free water losses, particularly when the ambient temperature is high.

The majority of cases of hypervolemic hypernatremia are iatrogenic in origin. Excessive sodium bicarbonate administration in the treatment of cardiac arrest or lactic acidosis is a common cause; each 50-ml ampule of sodium bicarbonate contains approximately 1000 mEq/liter of sodium. Another common example is hospitalized patients who receive isotonic saline without free water replacement of insensible water losses. Other iatrogenic causes include (1) accidental intravascular injection of hypertonic sodium chloride to induce abortions, (2) hypertonic formula fed to infants, and (3) dialysis solutions containing an excessive amount of sodium.

A variety of syndromes are associated with mineralocorticoid excess, including Cushing's disease, primary hyperaldosteronism, and congenital adrenal hyperplasia. In these disorders, sodium and water are retained, leading to an expanded ECF. The expanded ECF inhibits ADH release so mild water losses and subsequent mild hypernatremia result.

SELECTED READING

Conley SB: Hypernatremia. *Pediatr Clin North Am* 37 : 365, 1990.
Votey SR, Peters AL, Hoffman JR: Disorders of water metabolism: Hyponatremia and hypernatremia. *Emerg Med Clin North Am* 7 : 749, 1989.

39
Hyponatremia

DEFINITION

Hyponatremia is defined as a serum sodium concentration less than 135 mEq/liter. Sodium and its associated anions account for more than 95 percent of extracellular fluid (ECF) solute and are the major factors in determining serum osmolality. Osmolality, or tonicity, is defined as the concentration of plasma solutes (or osmoles) per kilogram of water. Effective osmoles such as sodium and glucose affect water movement into and out of cells. Overall, changes in sodium concentration reflect altered regulation of water, not changes in the body's sodium content alone.

The first step in determining the cause of hyponatremia is to calculate serum osmolality using the following equation:

$$\text{osmolality} = 2\text{Na}^+ \text{ (mEq/L)} + \frac{\text{glucose}}{18} \text{ (mg/dl)} + \frac{\text{BUN}}{2.8} \text{ (mg/dl)}$$

Where Na$^+$ = sodium concentration
BUN = blood urea nitrogen

Normal serum osmolality is 275 to 285; a value less than 275 is hypotonic while one greater than 285 is hypertonic. Causes of hyponatremia may be divided into three categories, based on the serum tonicity: (1) isotonic, (2) hypertonic, and (3) hypotonic.

ETIOLOGY
I. Isotonic
   A. Pseudohyponatremia (hyperlipidemia, hyperproteinemia)
   B. Isotonic infusions (glucose, mannitol)

II. Hypertonic
   A. Hyperglycemia (uncontrolled diabetes mellitus, total parenteral nutrition)
   B. Hypertonic infusions (glucose, mannitol)
III. Hypotonic
   A. Hypovolemia
      1. External losses (gastrointestinal, skin)
      2. Third-space losses (burns, pancreatitis)
      3. Renal losses (diuretics, renal damage)
      4. Adrenal insufficiency (Addison's disease, abrupt withdrawal of exogenous corticosteroids)
   B. Isovolemic
      1. Water intoxication
      2. Renal failure
      3. Sick-cell syndrome
      4. Oxytocin
      5. Syndrome of inappropriate antidiuretic hormone (SIADH)
   C. Hypervolemic
      1. Congestive heart failure
      2. Cirrhosis
      3. Nephrotic syndrome

DISCUSSION

The clinical manifestations of hyponatremia depend on the level of serum osmolality, its rate of change, and the etiology of the disorder. If patients have hypertonic hyponatremia, symptoms are usually attributable to (1) hyperglycemia or (2) the reason for administering mannitol, such as increased intracranial pressure. In isotonic states, symptoms are related to the effects of hyperlipidemia or hyperproteinemia. It is the patient with the hypotonic form who presents with the characteristic neurologic disturbances of hyponatremia, such as confusion, nausea, stupor, seizures, and coma. In these cases, if hyponatremia evolved slowly (over days to weeks), symptoms become apparent at a lower serum sodium level than if it developed acutely. Focal neurologic signs are unusual unless there is an underlying central nervous system disorder.

The first step in diagnosis is to calculate the serum osmolality. Although sodium and its associated anions are the major influence on ECF, other osmoles become a factor when present in large amounts. With hypertonic hyponatremia, an accumulation of effective osmoles (glucose, mannitol) in the ECF draws free water out of the cells, thereby diluting the sodium concentration. In general, each 100 mg/dl increase in serum glucose reduces the sodium concentration by 1.6 mEq/liter.

If the calculated serum tonicity is normal, serum lipid and protein levels should be measured. Both hyperproteinemia, as in multiple myeloma and Waldenström's macroglobinulemia, and hyperlipidemia can cause pseudohyponatremia (Fig. 39-1). In these disorders, large quantities of protein or lipid displace free water from the plasma. Each unit volume (e.g., 10 ml) of plasma contains less water and less sodium; however, the sodium concentration and osmolality in the remaining water remain normal. Since laboratories report sodium per liter of plasma, the value reported will be spuriously low. Infusions of isotonic glucose initially produce isotonic hyponatremia; glucose prevents water movement out of cells while free water dilutes the sodium concentration in the serum. As glucose is metabolized by cells, the free water remains and an isotonic becomes a hypotonic hyponatremia.

The last category, hypotonic hyponatremia, requires an assessment of the patient's volume status and urine sodium values. Edematous patients have hypervolemic hyponatremia. In these individuals, the effective blood volume is reduced, leading to enhanced renal sodium absorption and therefore low urinary sodium values. It develops late in the course of congestive heart failure or liver disease and may be worsened by aggressive treatment with diuretics.

Patients with hypovolemic hyponatremia have characteristic findings of dehydration including decreased skin turgor,

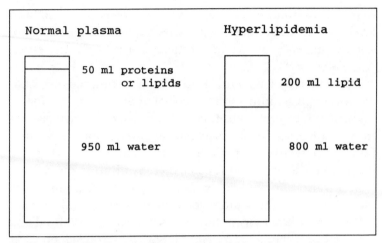

Figure 39-1. The normal plasma water volume has a sodium content of 150 mEq/L. However, the laboratory calculates sodium values based on 1000 ml, not 950 ml, of water. Therefore,

$$950 \text{ ml} \times 150 \text{ mEq/L} = \frac{142{,}500 \text{ mEq/L}}{1000 \text{ ml}} = \text{approximately 143 mEq/L}$$

If the same concentration is dissolved in 800 ml of plasma water, the laboratory value will be artificially low:

$$800 \text{ ml} \times 150 \text{ mEq/L} = \frac{120{,}000 \text{ mEq/L}}{1000 \text{ ml}} = 120 \text{ mEq/L}$$

tachycardia, and orthostatic hypotension. It is due to either (1) external losses from the kidneys or gastrointestinal tract or (2) redistribution from the plasma into interstitial spaces ("third-spacing"). Protracted diarrhea, vomiting, and naso-gastric suction are causes of gastrointestinal losses, while third-space translocation is due to burns, peritonitis, or pancreatitis. In these patients, urine sodium values are usually low. In contrast, patients with renal tubular damage or receiving diuretics will have an elevated urine sodium value. Patients with adrenal insufficiency have (1) sodium depletion due to aldosterone deficiency and (2) inappropriate anti-diuretic hormone (ADH) release due to cortisol deficiency.

Isovolemic hyponatremia is usually associated with mild water overload; however, since two-thirds of the water is intracellular, edema is not seen. The classic cause is SIADH, in which a patient has excessive release of ADH, leading to water retention. The release of ADH can be triggered by various pulmonary, central nervous system, cardiac, metabolic, or neoplastic disorders (Table 39-1). Common causes include narcotics, such as morphine, small cell carcinoma of the lung, and positive-pressure ventilation. SIADH is a diagnosis of exclusion; therefore, it is imperative that disorders of the kidney, adrenal glands, and thyroid are excluded before this diagnosis is made.

Other causes of isovolemic hyponatremia include renal failure in patients who are unable to excrete free water and

Table 39-1. Differential Diagnosis of the Syndrome of Inappropriate Antidiuretic Hormone (SIADH) Secretion

Neoplasms
   Lung (small cell in 80%), pancreas, duodenum, lymphoma,
      ureter, prostate, Ewing's sarcoma
Pulmonary
   Infection (viral, bacterial, fungal), abscess, asthma, respiratory
      therapy
Central nervous system
   Trauma, neoplasms, infections, vascular, degenerative diseases
      (including aging), psychoses
Cardiac
   Atrial tachycardias, post-mitral-commissurotomy syndrome
Metabolic
   Myxedema, adrenal insufficiency, acute porphyria
Stress
Drugs
   Hypoglycemic agents (chlorpropamide, tolbutamide),
      antineoplastic drugs (cyclophosphamide, vincristine),
      narcotics (morphine, barbiturates), psychotropics
      (phenothiazine derivatives)

Source: Narins RG, Krishna GG: Disorders of water balance. In Stein JH (ed): *Internal Medicine*, 3rd ed. Boston: Little, Brown, 1990. P 838.

sick-cell syndrome. Sick-cell syndrome, or reset osmostat, is a rare condition seen in disorders such as cirrhosis and pulmonary tuberculosis. It is characterized by a lower ECF osmolality that triggers ADH release, so that fluid is retained at a lower plasma osmolality value. Water ingestion alone rarely can overcome free water excretion mechanisms to produce hyponatremia.

SELECTED READING

Berry PL, Belsha CW: Hyponatremia. *Pediatr Clin North Am* 37 : 351, 1990.
Votey SR, Peters AL, Hoffman JR: Disorders of water metabolism: Hyponatremia and hypernatremia. *Emerg Med Clin North Am* 7 : 749, 1989.

40
Hyperkalemia

DEFINITION

Hyperkalemia is defined as a serum potassium (K^+) level greater than 5.5 mEq/liter. Since only 1 to 2 percent of total body potassium is found in the serum, an increase in serum K^+ does not imply an increase in total body stores. Causes of hyperkalemia can be divided into two categories based on whether the total amount of potassium in the body is normal or increased.

ETIOLOGY

I. Normal total body potassium
  A. Spurious (pseudohyperkalemia)
    1. Local K^+ release (tourniquet)
    2. Sample hemolysis
    3. Blood dyscrasias (thrombocytosis, leukocytosis)
  B. Decreased K^+ entry into cells
    1. Beta-adrenergic blocking agents (propranolol)
    2. Diabetes mellitus
    3. Autonomic insufficiency
  C. Increased K^+ loss from cells
    1. Hyperkalemic periodic paralysis
    2. Exercise
    3. Tissue catabolism (necrosis, injury)
    4. Acute acidosis (respiratory, metabolic)
    5. Drugs (digitalis poisoning, succinylcholine)
    6. Tumor lysis following chemotherapy (leukemia, lymphoma)

II. Excessive total body potassium
   A. Aldosterone deficiency/defect
      1. Adrenal insufficiency (Addison's disease)
      2. Hyporeninemic hypoaldosteronism
      3. Angiotensin-converting enzyme inhibitors (captopril, enalopril)
   B. Decreased responsiveness to aldosterone
      1. Renal failure
      2. Renal tubular disorders
      3. Potassium-sparing diuretics (triamterene, spirono-lactone)
   C. Administration of potassium-containing compounds (potassium chloride, potassium penicillin, salt substitutes)

DISCUSSION

Potassium is the most abundant intracellular cation, with a concentration of 150 mEq/liter. Changes in the serum K^+ levels lead to alterations in the intracellular-extracellular potassium ratio. Since potassium is the major factor determining transmembrane potentials, an increase in extracellular K^+ leads to partial depolarization of the cell membrane. The greatest impact is on the cardiac conducting system. When the potassium level rises above 6 mEq/liter, tall, peaked T waves develop on the electrocardiogram (ECG). As the level increases, the QRS complex lengthens, ultimately giving the ECG a "sine wave" appearance; this finding is soon followed by ventricular fibrillation or cardiac standstill. Other consequences of hyperkalemia include neuromuscular weakness and metabolic acidosis.

Potassium is excreted almost exclusively by the kidney. Patients with chronic hyperkalemia invariably have some degree of impaired renal function. In patients with normal renal function, extracellular increases in potassium can cause hyperkalemia if it occurs suddenly, as with intravenous administration of potassium-containing compounds.

Initially, spurious elevations in K^+ should be ruled out. These increases can be caused by tourniquet ischemia during phlebotomy (particularly when the fist was repeatedly clenched), in vitro hemolysis of the blood sample, or blood dyscrasias. The serum of a hemolyzed blood sample is usually pink from free hemoglobin. Marked thrombocytosis or leukocytosis can be associated with in vitro potassium release, as these blood components are unusually fragile.

A review of the patient's history and laboratory studies may be beneficial. Patients with diabetes mellitus or autonomic insufficiency may have decreased potassium entry into cells, particularly when challenged with an exogenous potassium load. Aldosterone, a potent mineralocorticoid produced by the adrenal cortex, causes sodium resorption and potassium excretion by the kidneys; a deficiency of this hormone, as occurs with both adrenal insufficiency and primary hypoaldosteronism, causes renal sodium wasting and potassium retention. Renal pathology, such as end-stage renal disease or renal tubular disorders (acute interstitial nephritis, postrenal transplantation), may present with hyperkalemia secondary to mineralocorticoid resistance. In postrenal transplant patients, hyperkalemia may be more common when cyclosporine is administered. In acute metabolic or respiratory acidosis, hydrogen ions move into cells in exchange for potassium ions. In these cases, the serum potassium level may be normal to high in spite of total body potassium depletion, a situation that occurs frequently in diabetic ketoacidosis. A rare cause of elevated serum K^+ is hyperkalemic periodic paralysis, an autosomal dominant disorder characterized by episodic hyperkalemia and muscle weakness or paralysis; the exact mechanism is unknown. Exhausting exercise may transiently increase K^+ up to 2 mEq/liter. Lastly, patients with large amounts of tissue catabolism, such as burns or trauma, or rapid tumor lysis following chemotherapy may have the sudden release of potassium from cells into the circulation.

Drugs cause hyperkalemia by a variety of mechanisms. Digitalis intoxication causes severe hyperkalemia by poisoning the sodium-potassium adenosine triphosphatase pump. Potassium-sparing diuretics, such as triamterene, amiloride, or spironolactone, inhibit the effect of aldosterone at the kidney, leading to potassium retention. Exogenous potassium loads can be given either directly (potassium chloride) or indirectly (potassium penicillin, salt substitutes); for example, every 1 million units of potassium penicillin contains 1.7 mEq of potassium. Beta-receptor blocking drugs prevent the movement of potassium into cells and may cause an exaggerated response to potassium supplements. Angiotensin-converting enzyme inhibitors, such as captopril or enalopril, decrease angiotensin II production and ultimately reduce aldosterone release from the adrenal cortex.

Succinylcholine has been known to produce hyperkalemia since the Vietnam War. Cardiac arrest following succinylcholine administration was first noted in patients with paraplegia or burns. Subsequently, it has been reported in patients with central nervous system disorders such as closed head injury or hemiplegia, major trauma, intra-abdominal abscesses, or on chronic bed rest. In patients with lower motor neuron lesions, this response is felt to be secondary to the extrajunctional spread of acetylcholine receptors and depolarization of the entire muscle membrane with rapid efflux of potassium. The period of time after injury when succinylcholine can be given safely is unknown. In normal individuals, succinylcholine can cause a transient increase in K^+ of 0.5 to 1.0 mEq/liter.

SELECTED READING

Brem AS: Disorders of potassium homeostasis. *Pediatr Clin North Am* 37 : 419, 1990.

Zull DN: Disorders of potassium metabolism. *Emerg Med Clin North Am* 7 : 771, 1989.

41
Hypokalemia

DEFINITION

Hypokalemia is defined as a serum potassium (K^+) level less than 3.2 mEq/liter. Potassium is the most abundant intracellular cation, with a concentration of 150 mEq/liter. However, since only 1 to 2 percent is extracellular, decreases in serum levels do not necessarily imply depletion of total body stores. Hypokalemia can develop with or without total body potassium depletion; if total body K^+ depletion occurs, it is secondary to one of three mechanisms: (1) decreased intake, (2) extrarenal losses, or (3) renal losses.

ETIOLOGY
 I. Without potassium depletion
   A. Pseudohypokalemia
   B. Increased entry into cells (redistribution)
      1. Exogenous insulin administration
      2. Catecholamine administration
      3. Beta-receptor agonists (terbutaline, ritodrine)
      4. Hypokalemic periodic paralysis
      5. Respiratory alkalosis
      6. Hypothermia
      7. Rapid cell proliferation (leukemia, lymphoma)
 II. With potassium depletion
   A. Decreased intake
      1. Total parenteral nutrition (TPN)
      2. Clay ingestion (geophagia)
   B. Extrarenal losses
      1. Diarrhea

    2. Laxative abuse
    3. Vomiting
    4. Nasogastric suction
    5. Profuse sweating
  C. Renal losses
    1. Normotensive
      a. Metabolic acidosis (renal tubular acidosis, carbonic anhydrase inhibitors)
      b. Metabolic alkalosis (vomiting, diarrhea)
      c. Bartter's syndrome
      d. Acute myelocytic leukemia
      e. Hypomagnesemia
      f. Drugs (diuretics, cisplatin, carbenicillin)
    2. Hypertensive
      a. Primary hyperaldosteronism
      b. Adrenogenital syndrome
      c. Exogenous mineralocorticoids (licorice)
      d. Renovascular hypertension
      e. Cushing's disease

DISCUSSION

Potassium is the major determinant of the cell's transmembrane resting potential. This electrical potential, which normally is around -90 millivolts, is determined by the ratio of intracellular (K^+i) to extracellular (K^+e) potassium.

$$\text{resting potential} = \frac{K^+i}{K^+e} = -90 \text{ millivolts}$$

Changes in the potassium level affect K^+e proportionally more than K^+i, resulting in alterations in the electrical charge of the cell membrane. For example, hypokalemia increases this ratio and hyperpolarizes the cell membrane; these changes primarily affect the heart and neuromuscular junction.

At the heart, hypokalemia leads to hyperpolarization of the cardiac conduction tissue. A K^+ level less than 3.0 mEq/liter leads to ST segment depression, T wave inversion, and the development of U waves on the electrocardiogram. As hypokalemia worsens, the QRS complex widens, and supraventricular and ventricular arrhythmias may develop. At the skeletal muscles, hypokalemia may precipitate cramps and weakness; if severe, paralysis and rhabdomyolysis may ensue. Other consequences of hypokalemia include reduced renal blood flow, impaired insulin and aldosterone secretion, and metabolic alkalosis.

The body's potassium level is controlled by several complex mechanisms. Transient decreases in serum levels are buffered by cellular stores, and normokalemia is maintained. However, changes in either volume status or acid-base balance can have a major impact on the serum potassium.

Sodium (Na^+) is the major determinant of the intravascular volume; maintenance of the intravascular volume is one of the primary objectives of the body. Any decrease is detected by volume sensors in the vascular tree, which activate the renin-angiotensin-aldosterone system. Aldosterone helps regulate extracellular fluid volume by increasing sodium resorption from the urine. To maintain electrical neutrality, K^+ is exchanged for Na^+, and K^+ is excreted in the urine. In addition, if large loads of sodium are presented to the distal tubules of the kidney, as occurs when a patient receives potent diuretics or carbenicillin, Na^+ is exchanged for K^+ and kaliuresis ensues.

The second factor affecting potassium is the acid-base balance. If a patient becomes alkalotic, extracellular K^+ is exchanged for intracellular hydrogen ions (H^+); hypokalemia develops without potassium depletion. If alkalosis becomes severe, K^+ levels in the renal tubule cells increase; K^+ is now lost in the urine as H^+ is resorbed, leading to true total body potassium depletion.

Potassium redistribution from the serum into cells is the primary mechanism for low K^+ without potassium depletion;

in these cases, hypokalemia usually resolves without K^+ supplementation. Causes of intracellular shifts include exogenous insulin, administration of beta-receptor agonists for asthma (terbutaline) or premature labor (ritodrine), hypothermia, respiratory alkalosis, and rapid cell proliferation (acute leukemias or Burkitt's lymphoma). Insulin administration may unmask severe hypokalemia in patients with diabetic ketoacidosis. Hypokalemic periodic paralysis is an uncommon familial disorder of unknown etiology characterized by transient episodes of muscle weakness due to acute potassium shifts into cells. Pseudohypokalemia occurs when acute leukemic cells absorb potassium from the serum when a blood sample is allowed to stand before separation; it is an in vitro, not an in vivo, phenomenon.

Total body potassium depletion occurs in most cases of hypokalemia. Decreased intake rarely affects K^+ due to the large intracellular stores. However, hypokalemia can develop in patients who either receive TPN without adequate supplements or have geophagia. Geophagia, or clay ingestion, is seen in some areas of the southern United States; clay binds potassium in the intestines, thereby preventing its absorption.

Extrarenal losses of potassium may be direct, as with diarrhea or laxative abuse, or indirect, due to volume depletion. Liquid stool may contain up to 40 to 60 mEq/liter of potassium. Villous adenoma, a premalignant tumor, can actively excrete potassium, leading to profound losses. When patients lose large volumes of fluid, as can occur with vomiting or nasogastric suction, hypovolemia triggers renal sodium resorption and subsequent potassium loss; in these cases, little K^+ is directly lost from the upper gastrointestinal tract, since the potassium concentration in gastric fluid is only 5 to 10 mEq/liter.

Most potassium wasting occurs through the kidney; the etiologies can be divided into normotensive or hypertensive disorders. Diuretics, which account for most cases of renal potassium wasting with normotension, lead to hypokalemia by two mechanisms: (1) causing a large sodium load to be presented to the distal tubules, ultimately leading to K^+ losses, and (2) producing volume contraction due to large fluid losses, which further contributes to potassium wasting. Other causes of hypokalemia with normotension include Bartter's syndrome, a rare disorder caused by hyperplasia of the juxtaglomerular apparatus, renal tubular acidosis, and drugs, such as cisplatin, gentamicin, and carbenicillin. Hypomagnesemia can be associated with hypokalemia that is resistant to potassium replacement until the magnesium deficit is corrected.

If hypertension and hypokalemia are present, either renovascular disorders or excessive mineralocorticoids are the underlying cause. Primary aldosteronism or adrenogenital syndrome leads to increased aldosterone secretion, which ultimately increases sodium resorption and potassium excretion. Exogenous mineralocorticoids such as sodium glycyrrhizinate, a compound found in chewing tobacco and some licorice, produce hypokalemia in a similar manner. Other causes of hypokalemia and hypertension include Wilms' tumor in children, renovascular hypertension, and Cushing's disease, due to adrenal carcinoma or ectopic adrenocorticotropic hormone production.

SELECTED READING

Brem AS: Disorders of potassium homeostasis. *Pediatr Clin North Am* 37 : 419, 1990.

Zull DN: Disorders of potassium metabolism. *Emerg Med Clin North Am* 7 : 771, 1989.

42
Hypercalcemia

DEFINITION

Hypercalcemia is defined as a serum calcium level greater than 10.5 mg/dl. An elevation in serum calcium is found in about 1 percent of routine laboratory screens of medical patients. Primary hyperparathyroidism and malignancies account for over 90 percent of all cases. The remaining causes of hypercalcemia can be divided into three categories: (1) nonparathyroid endocrine disorders, (2) medications, and (3) miscellaneous disorders.

ETIOLOGY

I. Primary hyperparathyroidism
   A. Parathyroid adenoma
   B. Parathyroid carcinoma
   C. Parathyroid hyperplasia
II. Malignancies
   A. Lytic bone lesions (breast, lung, multiple myeloma)
   B. Humoral peptides (squamous cell carcinoma of the lung, carcinoma of pancreas, ovary, kidney)
   C. Ectopic vitamin D production (T cell lymphoma)
III. Nonparathyroid endocrine disorders
   A. Hyperthyroidism
   B. Pheochromocytoma
   C. Other (adrenal insufficiency, pancreatic islet cell tumors)
IV. Medications
   A. Thiazide diuretics
   B. Vitamin D toxicity (vitamins, granulomatous disease)

    C. Lithium
    D. Estrogens
    E. Milk-alkali syndrome
  V. Miscellaneous causes
    A. Immobilization
    B. Total parenteral nutrition
    C. Renal disease (acute, chronic)
    D. Familial hypocalciuric hypercalcemia

DISCUSSION

The signs and symptoms of hypercalcemia will depend on the degree of calcium elevation, the rate of rise, and the underlying cause. When modestly increased, hypercalcemia may be an incidental finding on routine biochemical studies. As the level increases, patients may experience anorexia, constipation, polyuria, or depressed central nervous system function. The electrocardiogram will show a shortened Q–T interval. If hypercalcemia develops rapidly, signs and symptoms will occur at a lower calcium level than if it evolves over days to weeks. Elevated calcium in the presence of increased phosphate levels can produce metastatic calcifications throughout the body; the effects depend on the sites of the calcifications.

Primary hyperparathyroidism, one of the most common endocrine disorders, is characterized by excessive secretion of parathyroid hormone (PTH). The major actions of PTH are (1) mobilization of calcium from bones and (2) conservation of calcium by the kidneys. Primary hyperparathyroidism is diagnosed by measuring simultaneously collected serum calcium and PTH levels; the diagnosis is confirmed when an elevated calcium level is discovered in the presence of an inappropriately elevated PTH level. The majority of the patients (80–85%) have an isolated parathyroid adenoma, while the remainder have either generalized parathyroid hyperplasia or parathyroid carcinoma. There is a definite association of hyperparathyroidism with multiple endocrine neoplasia (MEN) syndrome, types I and II.

In addition to symptoms of hypercalcemia, patients with hyperparathyroidism may develop disorders of the bones and kidneys. The classic bone finding is osteitis fibrosa cystica, which is associated with bone pain, pathologic fractures, and characteristic findings on microscopic studies. Renal disorders include nephrolithiasis (kidney stones) and nephrocalcinosis (calcium phosphate crystals throughout the renal parenchyma).

Malignancies produce hypercalcemia by several mechanisms. The most common, lytic bone lesions, are produced by metastatic breast and lung carcinoma and multiple myeloma. Humoral peptides, such as ectopic PTH, can be secreted by squamous cell carcinoma of the lung and carcinoma of the pancreas, ovary, or kidney. Ectopic vitamin D is synthesized by certain T cell lymphomas.

A variety of medications can lead to hypercalcemia. The most common, thiazide diuretics, sensitize the kidney to PTH and result in decreased calcium excretion; it may take 2 to 3 months after the diuretic has been discontinued before the calcium level returns to normal. Lithium, estrogens, and milk-alkali combination can produce elevated calcium levels. Combining milk and absorbable antacids was once used as a treatment for peptic ulcers; this syndrome is rarely seen today, since nonabsorbable antacids are prescribed.

Vitamin D causes hypercalcemia by several mechanisms. Vitamin D toxicity can occur in patients taking large doses of vitamins over the course of several months. Granulomatous diseases, such as sarcoidosis, produce hypercalcemia secondary to exaggerated gastrointestinal sensitivity to vitamin D and increased gastrointestinal absorption of calcium; in these patients, PTH is suppressed. Ectopic vitamin D can be produced by some forms of lymphoma.

Nonparathyroid disorders of the endocrine system that lead to hypercalcemia include hyperthyroidism and pheochromocytoma. Minimal elevations in calcium, which occur in up to 25 percent of patients with hyperthyroidism, are probably secondary to rapid bone turnover. Pheochromocytomas are associated with MEN syndrome type II and hyperparathyroidism. Other rare causes include adrenal insufficiency and pancreatic islet cell tumors.

Several miscellaneous conditions contribute to elevated serum calcium levels. Immobilization produces hypercalcemia in the presence of other disorders of calcium metabolism, such as Paget's disease. Patients may have mild elevations in serum calcium levels with either (1) acute or chronic renal failure with secondary hyperparathyroidism or (2) excessive calcium supplements administered in total parenteral nutrition. Familial hypocalciuric hypercalcemia is a rare disorder often mistaken for primary hyperparathyroidism; it differs by being transmitted as an autosomal dominant trait and by having normal PTH levels.

SELECTED READING

Lynch RE: Ionized calcium: Pediatric perspective. *Pediatr Clin North Am* 37 : 373, 1990.
Olinger ML: Disorders of calcium and magnesium metabolism. *Emerg Med Clin North Am* 7 : 795, 1989.

43
Hypocalcemia

DEFINITION

Hypocalcemia is defined as a total serum calcium concentration less than 8.5 mg/dl. Calcium regulation is under the control of parathyroid hormone (PTH) and vitamin D. PTH has four effects: (1) mobilization of calcium from bones, (2) increased renal absorption of calcium, (3) increased intestinal absorption of calcium, and (4) activation of vitamin D. The actions of vitamin D include increasing calcium absorption in the intestines. Therefore, disorders that affect the amount of or the action of PTH or vitamin D, along with a variety of miscellaneous factors, can lead to hypocalcemia.

ETIOLOGY

  I. Parathyroid hormone
    A. Decreased levels (true hypoparathyroidism)
      1. Postsurgical
      2. Hypermagnesemia
      3. Neonatal hypocalcemia
      4. Other (radiation, chemotherapy, infiltrative disease)
    B. Decreased action
      1. Hypomagnesemia
      2. Pseudohypoparathyroidism
 II. Vitamin D
    A. Decreased levels
      1. Lack of exposure to sunlight

2. Malabsorption (postgastrectomy, small bowel disease, cathartics, primary biliary cirrhosis, post-hepatic obstruction)
   B. Decreased action
   1. Chronic renal failure
   2. Vitamin D–dependent rickets, type I
   3. Severe hepatocellular disease
   C. Resistance to vitamin D
   1. Vitamin D–dependent rickets, type II
   2. Anticonvulsant-induced osteomalacia
III. Miscellaneous
   A. Hypoalbuminemia (malnutrition, liver disease, nephrotic syndrome)
   B. Alkalosis
   C. Circulating free fatty acids
   D. Acute pancreatitis
   E. Acute release of intracellular phosphate (rhabdomyolysis, chemotherapy)
   F. Massive transfusion of citrated blood or fresh frozen plasma
   G. Osteoblastic metastases (breast, prostate carcinoma)

DISCUSSION

Evaluation of the patient with hypocalcemia includes a thorough history, physical examination, and laboratory studies. Initially, one should determine whether true hypocalcemia exists. Approximately 50 percent of calcium is bound to albumin in the serum, while the remaining 50 percent is ionized and represents the biologically active portion. If the albumin level is decreased, as in patients with severe malnutrition or nephrotic syndrome, the total serum calcium level will be depressed. In general, for every 1 g/dl reduction in albumin, the total calcium is decreased by 0.8 mg/dl. In these instances, the ionized calcium will usually be normal. When the ionized calcium is low (less than 1 mg/dl), true hypocalcemia exists.

The acid-base balance affects the amount of calcium bound to albumin; in alkalosis more calcium is bound, while less is bound with acidosis. A rise in pH of 0.1 unit decreases serum ionized calcium by 0.16 mg/dl; however, the total calcium remains unchanged. Circulating free fatty acids allow more calcium to bind to albumin, decreasing the ionized concentration. In these cases, an ionized calcium level should be measured.

Most of the symptoms of hypocalcemia are due to neuromuscular irritability and develop when the ionized calcium level is low. Initial features include cramps in the extremities and muscle weakness. As the levels become severely depressed, patients may experience tetany and convulsions. In neonates, hypocalcemia may first present as apnea. On physical examination, two findings that indicate hypocalcemia are Chvostek's and Trousseau's signs. Chvostek's sign is contraction of the facial muscles elicited by tapping the facial nerve. Trousseau's sign is produced by placing a tourniquet around the arm, leading to carpopedal spasm. Profound hypocalcemia also affects the heart, as it lengthens the Q–T interval; this prolongation can lead to torsades de pointes or polymorphic ventricular tachycardia.

Several conditions elicited from the history may lead to the diagnosis. Patients who have received massive transfusions of blood or fresh frozen plasma may have transient hypocalcemia secondary to calcium binding by citrate. Acute pancreatitis leads to release of lipase from the pancreas; lipase triggers fat necrosis, which promotes the formation of calcium soaps. The acute release of intracellular phosphates, which occurs after chemotherapy is given for rapidly proliferating tumors (leukemia, lymphoma), can result in calcium phosphate precipitation and hypocalcemia. Patients with osteoblastic metastases, primarily from prostate or breast malignancies, may present with hypocalcemia, as these lesions rapidly take up calcium from the serum.

Parathyroid hormone is the most important factor regulating serum calcium levels. A variety of disorders can decrease

PTH levels. The most common cause is the inadvertent removal of the parathyroid glands during a total thyroidectomy. Removal of a parathyroid adenoma for hyperparathyroidism will cause a transient decrease in PTH, since the remaining glands have been chronically suppressed. In neonates, immaturity of the parathyroid glands may cause a transient period of mild hypocalcemia during the first 3 weeks of life. Hypermagnesemia inhibits the parathyroid glands, and PTH secretion is diminished. Other rare causes of decreased PTH levels include idiopathic hypoparathyroidism, radiation to the head and neck, and infiltrative diseases involving the parathyroid glands, such as Wilson's disease or hemochromatosis.

Two conditions cause decreased bone response to PTH. The classic example is pseudohypoparathyroidism, a genetic disorder characterized by end-organ resistance to PTH. These patients have a distinctive physical appearance consisting of short stature, round faces, and a short neck; it is associated with seizures and mental retardation. Secondly, severe hypomagnesemia leads to hypocalcemia by diminishing PTH action on the bones; in this case, a normal calcium level cannot be attained until hypomagnesemia is corrected.

Disorders of vitamin D metabolism are common causes of hypocalcemia. Overall, a quantitative vitamin D deficiency is rare, since vitamin D is produced in large quantities by the skin when exposed to ultraviolet light. Decreased intake is unlikely, since milk is fortified with vitamin D; however, decreased absorption can occur. Vitamin D is fat soluble, and disorders that lead to bile salt deficiency (primary biliary cirrhosis, posthepatic obstruction) will impair its uptake. Patients with small bowel disease, such as tropical or nontropical sprue, can have vitamin D malabsorption, as can patients with excessive intake of cathartics.

Second, vitamin D may be present but defective; since the activation line for vitamin D is long, it is vulnerable to disruption at several points. The classic disorder, vitamin D–dependent rickets type I, is an inborn error of vitamin D metabolism that presents during the first year of life. Defective activation occurs in patients with severe hepatocellular or renal parenchymal diseases. Chronic renal failure leads to impaired production by the skin and decreased hydroxylation by the kidney; hypocalcemia is a common finding in patients with renal failure. In addition, these patients have elevated phosphate levels, which accelerate calcium entry into bones.

Last, patients may be resistant to the actions of vitamin D. Vitamin D–dependent rickets type II is a familial disorder of end-organ resistance. It may appear during infancy, childhood, or early adolescence. Osteomalacia can occur in patients receiving anticonvulsants, such as phenobarbital and phenytoin, especially when combinations are used. It appears to be due to induction of hepatic microsomal mixed function oxidase activity and a shortened half-life of vitamin D.

SELECTED READING

Lynch RE: Ionized calcium: Pediatric perspective. *Pediatr Clin North Am* 37 : 373, 1990.

Olinger ML: Disorders of calcium and magnesium metabolism. *Emerg Med Clin North Am* 7 : 795, 1989.

44
Hypermagnesemia

DEFINITION

Hypermagnesemia is defined as an elevation of serum magnesium levels above 2.4 mEq/liter. Since magnesium is readily excreted by the kidney, hypermagnesemia is extremely uncommon in the absence of impaired renal function. Causes of hypermagnesemia can be divided into two categories: (1) decreased renal excretion and (2) increased magnesium load.

ETIOLOGY

I. Decreased renal excretion
   A. Renal insufficiency
   B. Renal failure (acute, chronic)
   C. Hyperparathyroidism
   D. Adrenal insufficiency (Addison's disease)
   E. Hypothyroidism
   F. Lithium intoxication
II. Increased magnesium load
   A. Endogenous
      1. Diabetic ketoacidosis
      2. Severe tissue injury (burns, trauma)
   B. Exogenous
      1. Magnesium-containing laxatives and antacids
      2. Parenteral magnesium administration (preeclampsia)

DISCUSSION

Hypermagnesemia is rare in the absence of renal insufficiency. In fact, serum magnesium remains at normal levels
until the glomerular filtration rate (GFR) drops below 30 ml/
minute. Magnesium comes from both exogenous and endogenous sources. The primary exogenous contributors are
drugs. Severe tissue trauma is the main source of endogenous
loads, since the intracellular concentration of magnesium, the
second most abundant intracellular cation, is approximately
25 mEq/liter.

The clinical effects of magnesium are primarily on the neuromuscular junction and cardiac conduction system. When
serum levels exceed 4 mEq/liter, deep tendon reflexes are
abolished; following deep tendon reflexes is one way magnesium therapy for preeclampsia is clinically monitored. As levels progressively increase, patients experience lethargy,
skeletal muscle paralysis, hypotension, and electrocardiographic changes (prolonged P–R, Q–T, and QRS intervals).
Complete heart block or asystole may occur when serum levels
reach 15 mEq/liter. Hypermagnesemia potentiates the effects
of both depolarizing and nondepolarizing muscle relaxants.

Impaired renal excretion of magnesium is secondary to (1)
renal failure, (2) several endocrine disorders, and (3) lithium
toxicity. Renal failure leads to hypermagnesemia, since the
kidney is the primary site of magnesium elimination. Hyperparathyroidism, hypothyroidism, and adrenal insufficiency
can lead to impaired renal excretion. Parathyroid hormone
directly affects the loop of Henle and increases magnesium
resorption; this action is countered to some degree by the
magnesuric effect of hypercalcemia. Lithium intoxication
also increases magnesium resorption.

Magnesium-containing compounds can contribute to elevated magnesium levels when the GFR is decreased. The most
common sources are antacids (magnesium-aluminum compounds such as Maalox or Mylanta) and laxatives (magnesium citrate). Large doses of parenteral magnesium given to

women with preeclampsia or to alcoholics with nutritional deficits can produce hypermagnesemia even when renal function is normal. In women with preeclampsia, magnesium can cross the placenta, producing elevated levels in the neonate.

SELECTED READING

Ghoneim MM, Long JP: The interaction between magnesium and other neuromuscular blocking agents. *Anesthesiology* 42 : 545, 1975.

Olinger ML: Disorders of calcium and magnesium metabolism. *Emerg Med Clin North Am* 7 : 795, 1989.

45
Hypomagnesemia

DEFINITION

Hypomagnesemia is defined as a decrease in serum levels of magnesium below the normal range of 1.5 to 2.4 mEq/liter. The total body magnesium content is approximately 25 mEq/liter. While it is the second most abundant intracellular cation, only 1 percent is extracellular. Therefore, decreases in serum levels may not accurately reflect total body stores. The causes of hypomagnesemia can be divided into four major categories: (1) decreased intake, (2) renal losses, (3) gastrointestinal losses, and (4) internal shifts.

ETIOLOGY

I. Decreased intake
   A. Malnutrition (alcoholism, anorexia nervosa)
   B. Total parenteral nutrition
II. Renal losses
   A. Diuretics (furosemide, bumetanide, osmotic diuretics)
   B. Metabolic acidosis (ketoacidosis, lactic acidosis)
   C. Renal tubular disorders (diuretic phase of acute tubular necrosis, postobstructive diuresis, postrenal transplantation, renal tubular acidosis)
   D. Acute ethanol ingestion
   E. Hypercalcemia
   F. Hypophosphatemia
   G. Drugs (cisplatin, aminoglycosides)
   H. Hypoparathyroidism
   I. Aldosteronism
   J. Hyperthyroidism

III. Gastrointestinal losses
  A. Diarrheal states
  B. Malabsorption (ulcerative colitis, regional enteritis, short-bowel syndrome)
  C. Laxative abuse
  D. Prolonged nasogastric suction
IV. Internal shifts
  A. Intravenous glucose
  B. Insulin administration
  C. Refeeding after starvation
  D. Acute respiratory alkalosis
  E. Acute pancreatitis
  F. "Hungry bone syndrome"

DISCUSSION

Magnesium primarily affects the central nervous system, neuromuscular junction, and heart. Patients with hypomagnesemia may present with generalized weakness, tremor, hyperreflexia, clonus, and seizures. Cardiac effects include prolonged P–R or Q–T intervals and ventricular arrhythmias. Major neuromuscular and cardiac abnormalities occur with more severe deficits (75 to 100 mEq). Ventricular tachycardia in the presence of severe hypomagnesemia may be resistant to conventional therapy. Low serum magnesium levels can directly contribute to hypokalemia and hypocalcemia; the magnesium deficit must be corrected before adequate potassium and calcium replacement can be achieved. For parenteral replacement, 1 g of magnesium sulfate contains 8.12 mEq/liter of magnesium.

The initial step in diagnosis is to review the patient's history and medication record thoroughly. One of the most common causes of magnesium depletion is chronic alcoholism, due to either low intake or increased renal losses. Other causes of decreased intake include starvation, as in young females with anorexia nervosa, and inadequate magnesium supplements in total parenteral nutrition (TPN). In addition, glucose loads from either TPN or refeeding after starvation can cause shifts of magnesium into cells.

Historical findings that may be helpful in diagnosis include (1) history of intestinal disease or surgery, (2) resolving renal insult (acute tubular necrosis or postrenal transplantation), (3) prolonged nasogastric suction, and (4) recent parathyroidectomy. Intestinal disorders involving the terminal ileum (regional enteritis) contribute to diminished magnesium uptake, as this portion of the small intestines is the predominant site for gastrointestinal absorption. Any damage to the renal tubules is associated with large urinary losses, since the loop of Henle is the primary site for magnesium resorption in the kidney. Large nasogastric losses of fluid may contribute to decreased magnesium levels, since the magnesium concentration in upper gastrointestinal fluids ranges from 0.4 to 1.1 mEq/liter. Following parathyroidectomy for hyperparathyroidism, the skeletal system may rapidly take up magnesium (along with calcium and phosphate) as part of the "hungry bone syndrome."

Another common cause of hypomagnesemia is drugs. Loop diuretics, such as furosemide or bumetanide, are major contributors to renal magnesium wasting; osmotic diuretics also contribute to renal losses. High-dose aminoglycosides or cisplatin treatment for malignancies can damage the loop of Henle, leading to increased urinary losses. Chronic laxative abuse can result in large magnesium losses, since the magnesium concentration in the colon may be as high as 14 mEq/liter.

Several laboratory studies may indicate the cause of hypomagnesemia. Both hypercalcemia and hypophosphatemia inhibit magnesium resorption in the loop of Henle, leading to renal magnesium wasting. Organic compounds such as lactic acids or ketoacids can also increase renal losses. The effects of parathyroid hormone are variable; while this hormone's direct effect on the tubules is to promote magnesium resorption, hyperparathyroidism may indirectly produce magnesuria due to the more potent effects of hypercalcemia.

SELECTED READING

Olinger ML: Disorders of calcium and magnesium metabolism. *Emerg Med Clin North Am* 7 : 795, 1989.

Tweedle DEF: Electrolyte disorders in the surgical patient. *Clin Endocrinol Metab* 13 : 351, 1984.

46
Hypoglycemia

DEFINITION

Hypoglycemia is defined as the level at which glucose utilization exceeds glucose production. It is dependent not only on a specific laboratory value but also on the presence of characteristic symptoms. In general, a patient is considered to be hypoglycemic when the plasma glucose level drops below 50 mg/dl. Traditionally, hypoglycemia has been classified as postprandial or fasting. Causes of fasting hypoglycemia fall into two categories: (1) underproduction of glucose or (2) overutilization of glucose.

ETIOLOGY

I. Postprandial (reactive)
   A. Alimentary hypoglycemia (upper gastrointestinal surgery)
   B. Enzymatic defects (galactosemia, hereditary fructose intolerance)
II. Fasting
   A. Underproduction of glucose
      1. Hormone deficiencies (hypopituitarism, adrenal insufficiency, glucagon deficiency, growth hormone deficiency)
      2. Substrate defects
         a. Neonatal hypoglycemia
         b. Severe malnutrition
         c. Ketotic hypoglycemia of infancy
      3. Enzymatic defects (congenital deficiencies of glycogenic enzymes [glucose-6-phosphatase])

        4. Acquired liver disease
          a. Cirrhosis
          b. Hepatic congestion (congestive heart failure)
          c. Acute viral hepatitis
        5. Drugs (alcohol, salicylates, propranolol)
    B. Overutilization of glucose
        1. Hyperinsulinemia
          a. Exogenous insulin administration
          b. Insulinoma
          c. Sulfonylureas
          d. Insulin antibodies
          e. Newborn infants of diabetic mothers
        2. Appropriate insulin levels
          a. Extrapancreatic tumors (sarcomas, fibromas)
          b. Systemic carnitine deficiency
          c. Factitious hypoglycemia
          d. Oral hypoglycemic drugs (chlorpropamide)

DISCUSSION

Both a low serum glucose and clinical symptoms should be documented before a patient is diagnosed as having hypoglycemia. The symptoms of hypoglycemia can be divided into two categories: (1) excessive secretion of epinephrine due to sympathetic discharge triggered by falling glucose levels and (2) dysfunction of the central nervous system (CNS) due to cerebral glucose deprivation. The characteristic adrenergic symptoms include anxiety, tachycardia, palpitations, and diaphoresis. The magnitude of the symptoms is inversely related to the serum glucose level, and symptoms quickly clear following glucose administration. The second grouping is related to neuroglycopenia, since glucose is the primary fuel substrate for the CNS. The symptoms include headache, lethargy, and confusion and may proceed to coma or death. Seizures are more common in children than adults. It may take hours to days for these symptoms to resolve after the glucose level has returned to normal.

Postprandial or reactive hypoglycemia develops almost exclusively in patients who have had upper gastrointestinal surgery, such as a vagotomy or gastric resection. Presumably gastric emptying time is increased, which leads to brisk glucose absorption and insulin release. Since the glucose level falls more rapidly than the insulin level, hypoglycemia results. This condition can be diagnosed using an oral glucose tolerance test provided that (1) the symptoms are temporally related to the low glucose level and (2) they resolve with glucose administration. Other causes of postprandial hypoglycemia include rare enzymatic defects leading to hereditary fructose intolerance or galactosemia; these disorders become apparent in early childhood.

The majority of cases of hypoglycemia occur when patients are fasting and usually indicate a specific disease process. Causes of fasting hypoglycemia can be categorized according to the amount of exogenous glucose needed to prevent hypoglycemia over a 24-hour period. If more than 200 g is required, overutilization is the primary problem, since the daily hepatic production of glucose during fasting is sufficient to prevent hypoglycemia in normal individuals (100 to 200 g). In these cases, some degree of underproduction is also present. If hypoglycemia is prevented with less than 200 g of glucose, either underproduction or overutilization of glucose is the underlying problem.

Many of the reasons for underproduction of glucose can be identified by careful history and physical examination. During infancy the most common cause is decreased oral intake. Infants have immature livers and a reduced ability to store or to produce glucose. Combined with a higher resting metabolic rate, decreased intake, which occurs in neonates prior to elective surgery, can quickly lead to hypoglycemia. It commonly presents as lethargy or apnea. Other causes of hypoglycemia in infancy or early childhood include congenital deficiencies or defects of glycogenic enzymes. Glucose-6-phosphatase deficiency is the classic example, as glycogen stores in the liver are unable to break down into glucose. In addition, deficiencies in hepatic phosphorylase and glycogen synthetase affect glucose production.

A variety of acquired hepatic disorders and hormone deficiencies can cause underproduction of glucose. Hepatic congestion secondary to right-sided heart failure is particularly troublesome; cirrhosis or acute viral hepatitis can also interfere with glucose metabolism. Of the hormone deficiencies, hypopituitarism and adrenal insufficiency are the most common causes, while defects in glucagon secretion are rare.

A number of drugs can impair glucose production. The most common is ethanol, followed by salicylates (in children) and propranolol. As little as 25 mg/dl of alcohol can interfere with glucose production after a period of fasting when hepatic glycogen stores are depleted. Propranolol not only impairs the glycogenolytic response to hypoglycemia but also blunts the symptoms by blocking the adrenergic receptors' reaction to epinephrine.

Overutilization of glucose occurs when insulin levels are either high or normal and is usually due to drugs or tumors. Exogenous insulin often leads to hypoglycemia in diabetic patients who are not receiving adequate glucose loads. Surreptitious insulin administration may be mistaken for insulinoma, a tumor originating in the pancreas, since both are associated with high insulin levels. However, elevations in the C-peptide level, the connecting peptide cleaved from proinsulin during its conversion to insulin, indicate endogenous insulin hypersecretion, while low levels signify exogenous hyperinsulinemia. Rebound hypoglycemia can occur in newborn infants of diabetic mothers. The elevated glucose in the mother presents a constant load to the fetus who increases insulin secretion; when the glucose source is interrupted at birth, the elevated insulin levels persist, leading to hypoglycemia. Patients with insulin antibodies may develop hypoglycemia, although the exact mechanism is poorly understood. Sulfonylureas, which act as insulin secretagogues, can produce hypoglycemia.

Hypoglycemia in conjunction with normal insulin levels may indicate a solid extrapancreatic tumor. The majority are fibromas or sarcomas and usually have reached a large size before causing hypoglycemia. Oral hypoglycemics such as chlorpropamide can have a long half-life and exert their hypoglycemic effect after patients have been made NPO for surgery. Other causes of hypoglycemia with normal insulin levels include hepatomas and systemic carnitine deficiency.

SUGGESTED READING

Haymond MW: Hypoglycemia in infants and children. *Endocrinol Metab Clin North Am* 18 : 211, 1989.

Yealy DM, Wolfson AB: Hypoglycemia. *Emerg Med Clin North Am* 7 : 837, 1989.

47
Hypophosphatemia

DEFINITION

Hypophosphatemia is defined as a serum phosphate level less than 3.0 mg/dl. It is commonly encountered in clinical practice, with approximately 2 percent of all hospital admissions having low levels. Causes of hypophosphatemia fall into three categories: (1) decreased gastrointestinal absorption, (2) increased renal excretion, and (3) increased cellular uptake.

ETIOLOGY
I. Decreased gastrointestinal absorption
   A. Malnutrition
   B. Malabsorption (phosphate-binding antacids)
II. Increased renal excretion
   A. Primary hyperparathyroidism
   B. Secondary hyperparathyroidism
   C. Fanconi's syndrome
   D. Vitamin D–resistant rickets
   E. Diuretic phase of acute tubular necrosis
   F. Postrenal transplantation
   G. Glucosuria
   H. Idiopathic hypercalciuria
   I. Acetazolamide therapy
III. Increased cellular uptake
   A. Glucose-insulin infusions
   B. Catecholamine infusions
   C. Respiratory alkalosis
   D. Total parenteral nutrition (TPN)

E. "Hungry bone syndrome"
F. Alcohol withdrawal
G. Treatment of diabetic ketoacidosis

DISCUSSION

Inorganic phosphate has two important roles in the body: (1) formation of high-energy bonds (adenosine triphosphate) and (2) creation of 2,3-diphosphoglycerate (2,3-DPG). Depletion of high-energy bonds leads to the symptoms associated with hypophosphatemia, namely anorexia, muscle weakness, dizziness, and with severely depressed levels, encephalopathy. With acute depletion of phosphate, rhabdomyolysis and intravascular hemolysis may develop. Low levels of 2,3-DPG in erythrocytes may lead to tissue hypoxia secondary to impaired oxygen unloading at the cellular level.

By carefully reviewing the patient's history, most causes of hypophosphatemia can be uncovered. Low serum phosphate secondary to decreased oral intake is rare. Large quantities of aluminum or magnesium-containing antacids bind phosphates and render them unabsorbable. Primary and secondary hyperparathyroidism are the most common causes of renal phosphate wasting; secondary hyperparathyroidism is commonly seen in patients with end-stage renal disease. Renal disorders associated with hyperphosphaturia are Fanconi's syndrome, postrenal transplantation, and the diuretic phase of acute tubular necrosis. Hyperglycemia with glucosuria may promote renal phosphate excretion. Vitamin D–resistant rickets is a sex-linked dominant disorder that manifests itself in patients between 1 and 2 years of age. This condition causes impaired absorption of filtered phosphate. The clinical presentation varies from no symptoms to severe bone disease.

Increased cellular uptake is the most common cause of hypophosphatemia in hospitalized patients. Glucose-triggered insulin release promotes phosphate movement into cells from the extracellular pool. The combination of acute respiratory alkalosis and glucose infusions is frequently associated with low phosphate levels. Catecholamine infusions cause phosphate redistribution similar to the effects of insulin. Rapid uptake of phosphate during refeeding occurs commonly in chronic alcoholics or malnourished patients receiving TPN; hypophosphatemia may develop if phosphate supplements are inadequate. Patients with diabetic ketoacidosis may have profound depletion of total body phosphate secondary to glucosuria; treatment with insulin causes intracellular movement of phosphate and further depression of serum levels. "Hungry bone syndrome" occurs after correction of primary or secondary hyperparathyroidism; the rapid remineralization of bone can lead to severe hypophosphatemia.

SELECTED READING

Knochel JP: The pathophysiology and clinical characteristics of severe hypophosphatemia. *Arch Intern Med* 137 : 203, 1977.
Tweedle DEF: Electrolyte disorders in the surgical patient. *Clin Endocrinol Metab* 13 : 351, 1984.

VII
Hematologic

48
Bleeding

DEFINITION

Bleeding is defined as a breakdown in hemostasis. Intra-operative bleeding is most likely due to inadequate surgical hemostasis and impaired vascular integrity. Once this source has been excluded, the causes of bleeding can be categorized according to disorders of (1) platelets, (2) clotting factors, or (3) vessel walls.

ETIOLOGY

I. Platelets
  A. Quantitative—see Chapter 51
  B. Qualitative—see Chapter 52
II. Clotting factor deficiency/dysfunction
  A. Congenital (hemophilia A, Christmas disease)
  B. Acquired
    1. Liver disease
    2. Decreased vitamin K (malabsorption, hemorrhagic disease of the newborn)
    3. Anticoagulants (heparin, warfarin)
    4. Factor inhibitors (lupus anticoagulant, following factor VIII therapy)
    5. Primary fibrinolysis
    6. Secondary fibrinolysis (disseminated intravascular coagulation [DIC], drugs [streptokinase, urokinase])
    7. Massive blood transfusion
    8. Post–cardiopulmonary bypass coagulopathy (PCC)

III. Vessel walls
  A. Defective capillary walls (scurvy, Cushing's syndrome, senile purpura)
  B. Inflammatory (Henoch-Schönlein syndrome)

DISCUSSION

A thorough history and physical examination are the initial steps in diagnosis. Bleeding may be secondary to platelets if the count is low (idiopathic thrombocytopenic purpura, massive blood transfusion) or if the bleeding time is prolonged (patients on chronic aspirin therapy). Platelet disorders should be suspected when a patient has petechiae over the neck and upper torso. (See Chaps. 51 and 52.)

After platelet disorders have been excluded, defects in clotting factors should be evaluated. Laboratory tests are essential for diagnosis and should include a prothrombin time (PT) and partial thromboplastin time (PTT). The PT measures the function of the extrinsic clotting system, while the PTT determines the integrity of the intrinsic system (Fig. 48-1). Factor levels usually are severely depressed (less than 30% of normal) before the PT or PTT is prolonged. The thrombin time, a less commonly ordered test, is useful in detecting deficiencies in fibrinogen and the presence of fibrin degradation products.

Male patients with congenital bleeding disorders may have hemophilia A (classic) or hemophilia B (Christmas disease); both diseases are sex-linked hereditary disorders. Hemophilia A appears to be due to the production of normal amounts of nonfunctioning factor VIII, while hemophilia B is due to a deficiency of normal factor IX. After repeated treatment with factor VIII concentrates, patients may develop antibodies directed against this factor; these antibodies, or inhibitors, interfere with the function of further concentrate transfusions. In such cases, measuring levels of these inhibitors may be diagnostic.

Most causes of elevations of the PT or PTT are acquired. Liver disease is one of the most common causes of bleeding; patients with severe liver disease may have bleeding secondary to (1) decreased clotting factor production or (2) depressed clearance of fibrin degradation products (FDP). The synthesis of clotting factors is dependent on normal hepatocellular function and normal levels of vitamin K; derangements in either will result in depression of factor production. When decreased factor production is secondary to severe hepatocellular disease, cirrhosis is usually present. These patients have other stigmata of cirrhosis, such as ascites, asterixis, and esophageal varices.

The second cause of impaired factor synthesis is decreased levels of vitamin K. Vitamin K is essential for the synthesis of factors II, VII, IX, and X. It is produced by intestinal bacteria and green, leafy vegetables. Because of its lipophilic structure, vitamin K is absorbed only in the presence of bile salts. Bile salts may be decreased or absent with intrahepatic or posthepatic obstruction. Other causes of vitamin K deficiency include malabsorption syndromes and antibiotic "bowel preps," which eliminate normal bowel flora. Hemorrhagic disease of the newborn is due to low levels of vitamin K in the neonatal period. In these conditions, unlike hepatocellular disease, the PT and PTT can be corrected to normal by the parenteral administration of vitamin K.

Depressed clearance of FDP is an important contributor to bleeding in patients with liver disease. Several FDP fragments are potent anticoagulants. In healthy individuals, low levels of FDP normally produced are rapidly cleared by the liver. However, in patients with liver disease, not only are higher levels of FDP produced due to increased fibrinolytic activity, but also the levels rise further due to impaired removal from the circulation.

Other causes of prolonged PT and PTT include administration of anticoagulants, such as heparin or warfarin, or circulating anticoagulants. Patients with systemic lupus erythematosus may develop IgG antibodies against factor VIII; these antibodies, called lupus anticoagulants, generally

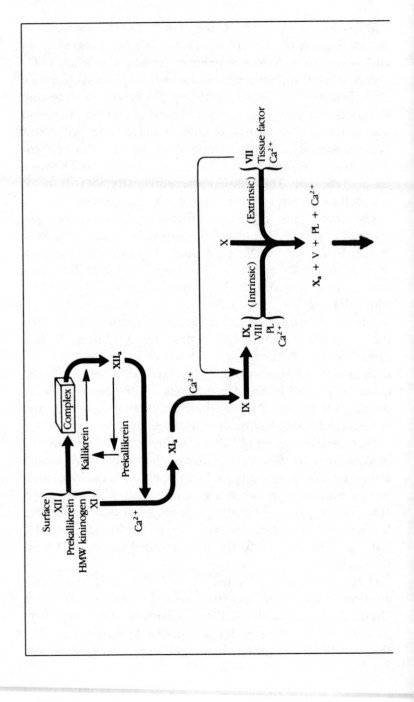

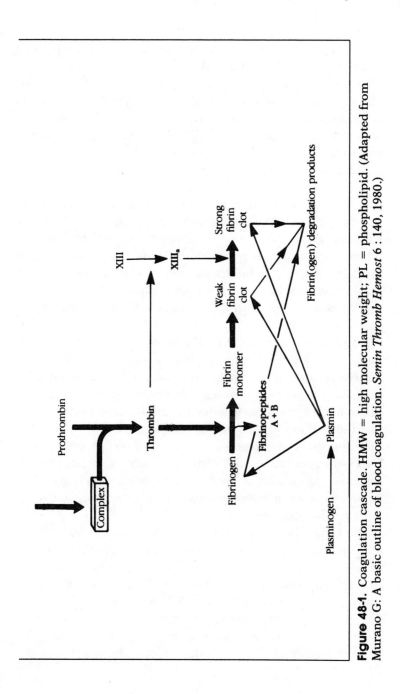

Figure 48-1. Coagulation cascade. HMW = high molecular weight; PL = phospholipid. (Adapted from Murano G: A basic outline of blood coagulation. *Semin Thromb Hemost* 6 : 140, 1980.)

do not cause clinical bleeding, unlike inhibitors of factor VIII in patients with hemophilia A.

Patients may have either primary or secondary fibrinolysis. The secondary form is the result of DIC or the administration of streptokinase or urokinase. DIC produces bleeding secondary to consumption of clotting factors and platelets and to production of FDP. DIC is seen in a variety of disorders, such as sepsis or transfusion reactions. Primary fibrinolysis is a rare disorder associated with cirrhosis or prostatic carcinoma.

Massive transfusions can lead to a coagulopathy primarily due to dilutional thrombocytopenia. Elevations of the PT or PTT can occur when the transfusion exceeds 10 units or when units of packed red blood cells instead of whole blood are administered. A mild elevation in the PT (less than 15 seconds) cannot be corrected with fresh frozen plasma since the PT of a unit of fresh frozen plasma is approximately 15 seconds.

A special situation is PCC. The causes of PCC are listed in Table 48-1. Once heparin has been adequately neutralized, platelet dysfunction is the leading cause of PCC. It is felt to be secondary to platelet degranulation produced by the cardiopulmonary bypass oxygenator. In addition to platelet dysfunction, dilutional thrombocytopenia may contribute to bleeding, even with levels as high as 100,000 platelets/mm^3. Excessive protamine administration may exacerbate bleeding, since protamine by itself is an anticoagulant. Other less common causes include dilutional clotting factor deficiencies, DIC, and fibrinolysis.

The third general category is bleeding due to vessel wall abnormalities. Although common, they usually do not cause serious bleeding problems. The mucous membrane or skin is primarily involved; bleeding starts immediately following injury, stops in less than 48 hours, and rarely recurs. The pathologic mechanisms involved are either impaired protein production for the capillary basement membrane, as in scurvy or Cushing's syndrome, or inflammation of the

Table 48-1. Causes of PCC

1. Unneutralized heparin
2. Platelet dysfunction
3. Thrombocytopenia
4. Coagulation factor deficiencies
5. Excessive protamine
6. Hyperfibrinolysis
7. Disseminated intravascular coagulation
8. Chronic coagulation disturbances—congenital or acquired

Source: Gravlee GP: Coagulation and anticoagulation: Problems during cardiac surgery. Excerpted from *38th Annual Refresher Course Lectures and Clinical Update Program* (1987), American Society of Anesthesiologists, 515 Busse Highway, Park Ridge, Illinois 60068-3189.

capillary wall, as in Henoch-Schönlein syndrome. In these cases, the PT, PTT, platelet count, and bleeding time are normal.

SELECTED READING

Cassady JF: Diagnosis and treatment of coagulopathy following cardiopulmonary bypass. *ASA Refresher Courses Anesthesiol* 18 : 85, 1990.

Glass D: Blood coagulation, coagulopathies, and anticoagulant therapy. *1990 Annual Refresher Course Lectures*. Lecture 162, pp 1–7.

Holahan JR: Coagulopathies. In Brady LL, Smith RB (eds): *Decision Making in Anesthesiology*. Toronto: Decker, 1987. Pp. 236–237.

49
Anemia

DEFINITION

Anemia is defined as a reduction in the normal number of red blood cells (RBCs) in the circulation. A hemoglobin level below 10 g/dl or hematocrit less than 30 percent has arbitrarily been defined as anemia. The causes of anemia can be divided into three categories: (1) decreased production, (2) increased destruction, and (3) loss of RBCs from the circulation.

ETIOLOGY

I. Decreased production
   A. Factor deficiency (iron, vitamin B_{12}, folic acid)
   B. Marrow failure
      1. Myelofibrosis
      2. Tumors (primary, metastatic)
      3. Toxic marrow suppression (lead, cancer chemotherapeutic agents, radiation therapy)
      4. Aplastic anemia
      5. Anemia of chronic disease (rheumatoid arthritis)
      6. Anemia secondary to end-stage renal disease
      7. Chronic liver disease
   C. Other (sideroblastic, thalassemias)
II. Increased destruction
   A. Autoimmune
      1. Disease-related (chronic lymphocytic leukemia [CLL], lymphomas, systemic lupus erythematosus)
      2. Drug-related (methyldopa, penicillin, quinidine)
      3. Other (paroxysmal cold hemoglobinuria)

B. Intravascular trauma (prosthetic heart valve, eclampsia, malignant hypertension, thrombotic thrombocytopenia purpura, disseminated intravascular coagulation [DIC], hemolytic-uremic syndrome, hemangiomas)

C. Membrane defect (sickle cell disease, hereditary spherocytosis, hereditary elliptocytosis, paroxysmal nocturnal hemoglobinuria)

D. Enzyme disorders (glucose-6-phosphate dehydrogenase [G-6-PD])

III. Loss from the circulation

A. Acute hemorrhage (trauma)

B. Chronic hemorrhage (menstrual, gastrointestinal)

C. Hematomas (retroperitoneal, acute epidural)

D. Hypersplenism

DISCUSSION

The first diagnostic step is determining whether the blood loss is acute or chronic. Acute loss, usually due to hemorrhage or hemolysis, is accompanied by tachycardia, orthostatic hypotension, pallor, and impaired mentation. If patients have underlying coronary artery disease, angina may be the initial manifestation of anemia; however, it is rare for anemia alone to produce angina in the absence of obstructive coronary artery lesions. If anemia has developed chronically, cardiovascular symptoms ordinarily are not present; the body has adapted to the low hematocrit by increasing both stroke volume and red blood cell 2,3-diphosphoglycerate to improve oxygen transport to the peripheral tissues.

A thorough review of the patient's history and medication record will often reveal the most likely etiology of the anemia. Individuals with end-stage renal disease have a baseline hematocrit of 25 to 27 percent due to impaired erythropoietin production, chronic blood loss (from hemodialysis and venipunctures), or both. A genetic or familial cause, such as sickle cell disease, thalassemia, hereditary spherocytosis, or G-6-PD deficiency, may be known. Chronic systemic diseases (e.g., rheumatoid arthritis) are associated with low-grade anemias secondary to marrow suppression by unidentified factors. Patients with cancer may have marrow failure due either to infiltration by tumor cells or to suppression by the cancer chemotherapeutic medications. Lead poisoning leads to anemia by several different mechanisms: (1) decreased erythrocyte production, (2) increased destruction, and (3) impaired hemesynthesis. It occurs in children who ingest lead paint found in older homes or apartments, particularly in inner city areas. Often the initial presentation is abdominal tenderness. Heavy menstrual periods or chronic gastrointestinal blood loss produce iron-deficiency anemia, while dietary folic acid deficiency is the primary cause of anemia in chronic alcoholics. Vitamin B_{12} deficiency occurs in patients with pernicious anemia and may develop following resection of the terminal ileum, the site of B_{12} absorption. Patients may have increased RBC destruction due to mechanical factors (malfunctioning prosthetic heart valves, DIC) or autoimmune disorders. The latter includes patients with lymphomas, CLL, or those receiving drugs known to produce autoimmune hemolytic anemia (e.g., penicillin, methyldopa, or quinidine). Infants with acute epidural hematomas may lose large amounts of blood into the cranium, leading to anemia and shock.

Diagnostic studies that are beneficial will depend on the historical findings. A complete blood count may reveal pancytopenia consistent with aplastic anemia or myelofibrosis. A review of the peripheral smear may show fragmented or damaged red blood cells, as seen when there is intravascular hemolysis or trauma. Patients with DIC will have the additional laboratory findings of prolonged coagulation times and depressed platelet levels. In these cases, the urine may have a pink color secondary to free hemoglobin from intravascular hemolysis, and serum chemistries will show an unconjugated hyperbilirubinemia. Examination of the stool for blood may reveal the gastrointestinal tract as the source of chronic blood loss. Other specialized studies that may be ordered include serum haptoglobin, serum iron, folic acid, and vitamin B_{12} levels, bone marrow examination, and cold and warm immunoglobulins.

A problem arises in diagnosing the degree of anemia in patients with acute hemorrhage, such as trauma victims. The initial peripheral blood sample may not show a drop in hematocrit, since both RBCs and plasma are lost. Under normal circumstances, it takes approximately 24 hours for equilibration to occur. However, if a patient is resuscitated with crystalloid solutions, thereby replacing the plasma volume, the hematocrit will reveal the magnitude of the blood loss sooner. If a pulmonary artery catheter is present, a mixed venous oxygen saturation will indicate whether there is adequate oxygen delivery to the tissues.

SELECTED READING

Beutler E: The common anemias. *JAMA* 259 : 2433, 1988.
Zauder HL: Preoperative hemoglobin requirements. *Anesthesiol Clin North Am* 8 : 471, 1990.

50
Polycythemia

DEFINITION

Polycythemia is defined as an increase in the total number of red blood cells (RBCs) in the circulation. Hematocrits greater than 55 percent in men and 50 percent in women are considered polycythemic. Polycythemia can be divided into two general categories, based on either an absolute or relative increase in the percentage of RBCs in the circulation.

ETIOLOGY

I. Absolute (increased red blood cell number)
   A. Primary—polycythemia rubra vera
   B. Secondary
      1. Hypoxemia (high altitude, pulmonary disease, cyanotic congenital heart disease, alveolar hypoventilation)
      2. Abnormal hemoglobin (congenital methemoglobinemia, carboxyhemoglobin, high-affinity variants)
      3. Hormone effects
         a. Inappropriate increases in erythropoietin (renal cell carcinoma, hemangioblastomas, hepatomas)
         b. Excessive corticosteroids
II. Relative (decreased plasma volume)
   A. Diuretics
   B. Dehydration
   C. Overtransfusion with packed red blood cells

DISCUSSION

The first step is to distinguish between absolute and relative polycythemia. Absolute polycythemia is the true increase in the total RBC mass due to an increase in RBC number. Relative polycythemia occurs when the concentration of RBCs increases due to the loss of plasma; in this form, the RBC mass may or may not be increased. The latter is usually due to dehydration, such as when patients have received diuretics (e.g., furosemide or mannitol) or bowel cleansing preparations without adequate volume replacement. A less common cause is the overtransfusion of packed RBCs; the hematocrit of one unit of packed RBCs is approximately 70 percent.

Absolute or true polycythemia can be divided into two types, primary and secondary. Primary polycythemia, also known as polycythemia rubra vera, is a myeloproliferative disorder characterized by erythrocytosis, thrombocytosis, leukocytosis, hyperuricemia, and splenomegaly. It occurs in individuals in later life (60 to 70 years old). When the diagnosis is in question, specialized studies, such as bone marrow examinations, plasma leukocyte alkaline phosphatase, or measurement of RBC mass using chromium-51 RBC isotope dilution, can be ordered.

Secondary causes of polycythemia account for the majority of cases. The underlying pathology is chronic tissue hypoxia. It appears that low oxygen saturation, rather than low arterial PO_2, is more important in triggering increased erythropoietin production. The highest hematocrits are seen in patients with congenital heart disease with right-to-left shunts, where they may reach 65 to 70 percent. The most common cardiac cause is tetralogy of Fallot, followed by transposition of the great vessels and tricuspid atresia. Other causes, such as chronic pulmonary diseases, living at high altitudes, and obesity-hypoventilation (pickwickian) syndrome can lead to increased RBC mass due to decreased or impaired oxygen transport from the alveoli to the blood.

Abnormal hemoglobins that are unable to unload oxygen at the tissues are another cause of chronic tissue hypoxia. These forms include (1) high-affinity variants transmitted as autosomal dominant traits (hemoglobin Chesapeake, hemoglobin Yakima), (2) methemoglobinemia, (3) carboxyhemoglobin (as occurs chronically in cigarette smokers), and (4) sulfhemoglobinemia. In these forms, the platelet and white blood cell counts are normal to slightly elevated.

A third cause of secondary polycythemia is due to increase in corticosteroids or erythropoietin. Both Cushing's syndrome and administration of large quantities of exogenous corticosteriods can stimulate erythropoiesis. Renal tumors (renal cell carcinomas, adenomas) and infratentorial brain tumors (primarily hemangioblastomas) can lead to an increase in erythropoietin and subsequent erythrocytosis; however, erythrocytosis secondary to tumors is extremely rare.

SELECTED READING

Barabas AP: Surgical problems associated with polycythaemia. *Br J Hosp Med* 23 : 289, 1980.

Oh W: Neonatal polycythemia and hyperviscosity. *Pediatr Clin North Am* 33 : 523, 1986.

51
Thrombocytopenia

DEFINITION

Thrombocytopenia is defined as a decrease in the number of platelets in the systemic circulation. The normal count varies between 150,000 and 400,000 platelets/mm^3; thrombocytopenia exists when the count is less than 100,000 mm^3. The etiology of thrombocytopenia can be divided into three categories: (1) decreased platelet production, (2) increased destruction, and (3) miscellaneous causes.

ETIOLOGY

I. Decreased platelet production
   A. Congenital (Chédiak-Higashi anomaly, Wiskott-Aldrich syndrome, Fanconi's syndrome)
   B. Acquired
      1. Aplastic anemia
      2. Cancer chemotherapy (myelosuppressive drugs)
      3. Radiation therapy
      4. Bone marrow infiltration (tumor, fibrosis)
      5. Drugs (alcohol, thiazides, estrogens)
      6. Viral infections
      7. Nutritional deficiencies (folic acid, vitamin B$_{12}$)
      8. Paroxysmal nocturnal hemoglobinuria
II. Increased platelet destruction
   A. Disseminated intravascular coagulation (DIC)
   B. Thrombotic thrombocytopenic purpura (TTP)
   C. Hemolytic-uremic syndrome

D. Drug-induced (gold salts, cimetidine, quinidine, heparin)
E. Autoimmune (idiopathic thrombocytopenic purpura [ITP], chronic lymphocytic leukemia [CLL], systemic lupus erythematosus [SLE])
F. Infection (viral, bacterial, mycobacterial)
G. Extracorporeal circulation
H. Giant cavernous hemangioma (Kasabach-Merritt syndrome)
I. Prosthetic heart valves
J. Preeclampsia (toxemia of pregnancy)
III. Miscellaneous
A. Splenic sequestration (congestive, infiltrative, neoplastic)
B. Massive transfusions

DISCUSSION

The first step is to determine whether the disorder is limited to platelets alone or if other blood studies are affected. Therefore, complete blood count (CBC), prothrombin time (PT), partial thromboplastin time (PTT), and renal and hepatic function tests should be obtained. If the red and white blood cell counts are normal, factors that cause generalized bone marrow suppression (aplastic anemia, cancer chemotherapy, radiation therapy, viral infections, bone marrow infiltration) are virtually eliminated. Elevated PT and PTT are seen in conjunction with massive transfusions of packed red blood cells and DIC. Patients who have received large quantities of packed red blood cells will develop a dilutional thrombocytopenia. The peripheral blood smear may show fragmented red blood cells, as occurs with DIC, TTP, or malfunctioning prosthetic heart valves. TTP is also associated with elevated renal function tests, neurologic deficits, and anemia. Hemolytic-uremic syndrome occurs in children younger than 6 years old and usually follows a minor febrile illness. It is characterized by fever, renal failure, anemia, and thrombocytopenia.

A review of the patient's history and medication record may give additional insights into potential causes of thrombocytopenia. Congenital causes of increased platelet destruction include Fanconi's syndrome and Chédiak-Higashi anomaly. Patients with CLL or SLE may develop autoantibodies against platelets. Drugs may induce thrombocytopenia either by immune mechanisms (quinidine, sulfonamides) or by direct toxic reaction to the bone marrow (cimetidine, gold salts). Chronic alcoholics may have (1) nutritional deficiencies of folic acid or vitamin B_{12}, (2) hypersplenism and subsequent platelet sequestration due to portal hypertension, or (3) direct marrow suppression secondary to alcohol. Patients with severe infections produced by staphylococci or streptococci may have increased platelet destruction due to release of exotoxins. Women in the third trimester of pregnancy may develop toxemia, with thrombocytopenia being a cardinal feature.

One of the most common causes of isolated thrombocytopenia is ITP. ITP is an autoimmune disorder characterized by purpura over the chest, neck, and limbs. While an acute form is most common in children 2 to 6 years old, a chronic recurrent form occurs most often in women 20 to 40 years old. The disease is usually controlled by administering corticosteroids or vincristine. However, many patients require splenectomy to remove the site of platelet destruction. In these patients, the steroid dosage should be raised prior to surgery to help increase the platelet count. If thrombocytopenia is severe, preoperative platelet transfusions should be considered.

SELECTED READING

Miller RD, Robbies TO, Tong MJ, Barton SL: Coagulation defects associated with massive transfusions. *Ann Surg* 174 : 794, 1971.

Reed RL II, Ciavarella D, Heimbach DM, et al: Prophylactic platelet administration during massive transfusion: A prospective, randomized, double-blind clinical study. *Ann Surg* 203 : 40, 1986.

Warkentin TE, Kelton JG: Heparin and platelets. *Hematol Oncol Clin North Am* 4 : 243, 1990.

52
Platelet Dysfunction

DEFINITION

The function of the coagulation system depends not only on an adequate platelet count but also on normal platelet activity. When a qualitative defect is present, the platelets may not react in the clotting process, even when present in sufficient numbers. The causes of platelet dysfunction can be divided into congenital and acquired disorders.

ETIOLOGY

I. Congenital
   A. Von Willebrand's disease
   B. Bernard-Soulier (giant platelet) syndrome
   C. Thrombasthenia (Glanzmann's disease)
   D. Thrombocytopathic purpura (platelet factor 3 deficiency)
II. Acquired
   A. Drug-induced (aspirin, nonsteroidal anti-inflammatory drugs [NSAIDs])
   B. Uremia
   C. Dysproteinemia (multiple myeloma, macro-globulinemia)
   D. Cirrhosis
   E. Myeloproliferative disorders
   F. Post–cardiopulmonary bypass

DISCUSSION

A qualitative defect in platelet function may be suspected when (1) bleeding continues in the presence of normal coagulation tests and platelet count, (2) the patient has been receiving a drug known to inhibit platelet function, or (3) there is a positive family history of a bleeding disorder. Physical findings include oozing from mucosal surfaces, from subcutaneous tissues, or around suture holes.

The first step in diagnosis is to obtain a template bleeding time. This study is performed by placing a 9-mm long by 1-mm deep incision on the forearm and then determining the length of time required for bleeding to stop; a normal bleeding time is less than 10 minutes. Clot retraction can be measured since platelets play a major role in this process; however, this test is not useful in the acute situation, as it takes 24 hours to complete. Other tests of platelet function are designed to evaluate and categorize the specific platelet abnormality; these specialized studies include measuring platelet release factor, platelet aggregation (adenosine diphosphate, collagen), and platelet adhesion.

Congenital causes of platelet dysfunction are rare except for von Willebrand's disease. Von Willebrand's disease is a hemorrhagic disorder transmitted as an autosomal dominant trait. It is heterogenous both in the severity of bleeding and in the underlying abnormality causing the bleeding. However, the cardinal feature is a prolonged bleeding time. Other diagnostic studies include measuring antihemophilic factor activity and platelet aggregation.

More commonly, functional platelet disorders are acquired. Drugs, primarily aspirin and NSAIDs, are the most common culprits. Aspirin irreversibly inhibits cyclooxygenase, thereby blocking thromboxane A_2 production and subsequent platelet aggregation. These effects persist for the life span of the platelets and may prolong the bleeding time for up to 1 week following a single dose of aspirin. NSAIDs also inhibit platelet function, although the effects usually resolve when the drug is discontinued. Compounds such as dextran impair platelet aggregation and increase the bleeding time by physically coating the platelets.

Acquired systemic diseases can directly affect platelet activity. Uremia is associated with generalized bleeding from mucosal surfaces and subcutaneous tissues; this dysfunction is partly reversed by adequate dialysis. Patients with cirrhosis and myeloproliferative disorders can have functional defects, the exact nature of which is unclear. Patients with dysproteinemias, such as multiple myeloma and macroglobulinemia, may have a prolonged bleeding time; it is thought that the abnormal globulin coats the platelet's surface, thereby interfering with normal function.

Last, a common acquired cause is post–cardiopulmonary bypass (CPB). Once heparin has been adequately neutralized, platelet dysfunction is the primary cause of post–CPB coagulopathy. The incidence varies with the type of oxygenators used (bubble versus membrane) and other components of CPB. The major defects are thought to be either degranulation of platelets or damage to the platelet membrane. It is felt that bubble oxygenators produce more platelet damage than membrane oxygenators, although the significance is reduced when the pump run is short (less than 2 hours). Treatment is controversial; however, desmopressin (DDAVP), which promotes release of von Willebrand's factor from the reticuloendothelial system, may be beneficial.

SELECTED READING

Addonizio VP: Platelet function in cardiopulmonary bypass and artificial organs. *Hematol Oncol Clin North Am* 4 : 145, 1990.

Spiess BD: Coagulation function in the operating room. *Anesthesiol Clin North Am* 8 : 481, 1990.

VIII
Equipment Errors

53
Pulse Oximetry

Theodore J. Heyneker

DEFINITION

Determination of hemoglobin saturation through noninvasive techniques has a history dating back over 100 years; however, only in the past decade have clinically useful pulse oximeters become available. As with any new clinical measuring device, there exists the potential for data to be misleading. To understand these shortcomings, a brief and simple look at the physics of this instrument is required.

The absorption of transmitted light is the mechanism on which pulse oximetry is based. Modern pulse oximeters transmit two wavelengths, 660 nm (visible red) and 940 nm (infrared). A light-emitting diode (LED) is the source of the transmitted light, while a photodiode is the detector. Light absorption by hemoglobin is species-unique and varies according to the transmitted wavelength (i.e., while hemoglobin "x" absorbs more light at 660 nm than hemoglobin "y," the reverse may be true at 940 nm). According to Beer's law, the absorption of light by a solution varies as a function of the concentration of the solute and the depth of the solution (or the distance through which the light is transmitted). If a known wavelength is transmitted through a known distance of a given solution, with a known absorption coefficient, the concentration of the solute can be obtained.

Determining hemoglobin concentration is complicated by the existence of four hemoglobin species: oxyhemoglobin (O_2Hb), reduced hemoglobin (Hb), carboxyhemoglobin (COHb), and methemoglobin (MetHb). To measure all four would require four transmitted light wavelengths, since according to Beer's law a different wavelength is required for each unknown concentration. Clinically used pulse oximeters employ only two wavelengths. Since carboxyhemoglobin and methemoglobin exist in very low concentrations except in rare situations, saturation measurements use only two species of hemoglobin. This measurement of "oxygen saturation" is referred to as the functional hemoglobin saturation:

$$\text{Functional saturation} = \frac{100 \ O_2Hb}{(Hb + O_2Hb)}$$

This is in contradistinction to the fractional hemoglobin saturation, which is the ratio of oxyhemoglobin to total hemoglobin.

$$\text{Fractional saturation} = \frac{100\% \times O_2Hb}{Hb + O_2Hb + COHb + MetHb}$$

The "depth of solution" is referred to as the DC component, which is composed of bone, muscle, skin, pigmentation, and nonpulsatile blood flow. Absorption during pulsatile flow, which is presumed to be arterial blood, is defined as the AC component (Fig. 53-1). Measurement of the transmitted light for two wavelengths is made during both the DC and AC phases. Using known absorption coefficients, the respective concentrations of the two hemoglobin species are determined. A ratio (R) of pulse-added absorbances is then made. (Distance is factored out, since distance or depth of solution is essentially the same for all measurements.)

$$R = \frac{AC\ 660/DC\ 600}{AC\ 940/DC\ 940}$$

The R wave is then correlated with data from normal volunteers on whom arterial oxygen saturation (SaO_2) readings

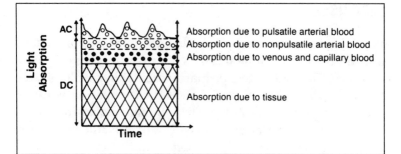

Figure 53-1. Schematic illustration of the light absorption through living tissue. Note that the AC signal is due to the pulsatile component of the arterial blood, while the DC signal is composed of all the nonpulsatile absorbers in the tissue: nonpulsatile arterial blood, venous and capillary blood, and all other tissues. (Adapted from Ohmeda Pulse Oximeter Model 3700 Service Manual, 1986, p 22.)

have been made. Overall, causes of errors in pulse oximetry fall into one of three categories: (1) changes in the AC component, (2) changes in the DC component, or (3) miscellaneous.

ETIOLOGY

I. Changes in the AC component
   A. Vasoconstriction (hypovolemia, hypotension, hypothermia, vasoconstricting medications)
   B. Motion
II. Changes in the DC component
   A. Increased levels of nonmeasured hemoglobins (methemoglobin, carboxyhemoglobin)
   B. Intravenous dyes (methylene blue, indocyanine green, indigo carmine)
   C. Skin or fingernail pigmentation
III. Miscellaneous
   A. Manufacturer programming
   B. Ambient light
   C. Variations in cardiac rate and rhythm
   D. Reuse of disposable equipment

DISCUSSION

Physiologic disorders can cause changes in the AC component and are the most common causes of errors in pulse oximetry readings. These disorders primarily are: (1) hypovolemia, (2) hypotension, (3) hypothermia, and (4) use of vasoconstrictor drugs, such as phenylephrine. The common underlying mechanism is vasoconstriction-induced loss of pulsatile flow; with pulselessness, SaO_2 is either underestimated or unreadable. However, the state of blood flow to vital organs cannot be assumed simply by the presence of a functioning pulse oximeter, since flows as low as 9 percent of normal can generate a pulse oximeter reading.

Motion artifact induced by patient's movement or shivering results in erroneous AC/DC ratios as a result of blood moving into and out of the digits. The resultant pulse oximeter saturation reading (SpO_2), if present at all, will not be reliable. Since the pulse oximeter can sample data for various preset time intervals, choosing a longer time-averaging mode may minimize the effects of motion at the expense of slowing the detection time for acute desaturations.

Multiple factors can affect the DC component. Methemoglobin and carboxyhemoglobin in significant levels cause an overestimation of SpO_2. When dyes are added to the blood, the ratio (R) of the pulse-added absorbances can be altered, resulting in erroneous SpO_2 reading. Significant desaturation to SpO_2 65 for 120 seconds has been reported using methylene blue. Lesser effects were noted for indocyanine green and indigo carmine. Surface dyes such as nail polish, especially red-brown colors, can reduce transmitted light, thereby affecting the SpO_2 reading. Placing the probe side-to-side on the finger will avoid this problem. More exotic dyes, such as the Middle Eastern coloring of the digits with henna, will limit access sites. Alternatives involve placing an ear clip on the ear or the lip. (In the latter case, the finger portion of a clear vinyl glove placed over the probe will preclude patient-to-patient contamination if the probe is reused.)

The calibration algorithms used by the pulse oximeter are only as good as the data from which they are derived (healthy volunteers under stable conditions). Comparison of pulse oximeters from six manufacturers has found significant variations of mean readings taken during acutely induced hypoxic plateaus. Ear probes were more accurate than finger probes due to the shorter lag time required for ear probes to reflect acute changes in SaO_2.

Ambient light sources can result in false readings. A normal SpO_2 has been recorded in a cyanotic child whose pulse oximeter probe was directly under an operating room light. Infrared heat lamps can also prevent the pulse oximeter from determining SpO_2. In an attempt to avoid this problem, most pulse oximeters are programmed to have the red and infrared LEDs fire alternately, enabling the photodiode to absorb each wavelength separately. This also enables the ambient light to be detected at intervals when neither LED is firing. The computer then subtracts the ambient reading. Xenon operating lamps have a rapid pulsatile quality that can confound the preprogrammed ambient light-detecting ability of the pulse oximeter. Likewise, very powerful external light sources such as infrared heating lamps, bilirubin lights, and sunlight can overpower the photodiode and preclude it from measuring the LED transmitted signal. Opaque shielding of the probe circumvents this problem.

It is generally assumed that a correct pulse oximeter heart rate is a requirement for accurate SpO_2, since this implies that the pulse oximeter is detecting cardiac-generated pulses. It has been noted in situations of pronounced dichrotic notches or irregular heart rates the pulse oximeter heart rate may be incorrect. However, the SpO_2 reading, if present, may be correct.

Reuse of disposable neonatal pulse oximeter probes (Nellcor Oxisensor Model N-25) has been reported to induce spuriously low SpO_2 readings. As a result of repeated use, the adhesive from the bandage-like portion of the probe can move, partially covering the LED and photodiode. Consequently, emitted and detected light intensities are decreased.

SELECTED READING

Severinghaus J: Oximetry: What does it tell you? *42nd Annual Refresher Course Lectures and Clinical Update Program.* American Society of Anesthesiologists. Lecture 266, pp 1–7.

Tremper KK, Barker SJ: Pulse oximetry. *Anesthesiology* 70 : 98, 1989.

54
Pulmonary Artery Catheter
Theodore J. Heyneker

DEFINITION

The pulmonary artery catheter is used to measure pulmonary artery occlusion pressure (PAOP). The PAOP estimates left ventricular end-diastolic pressure (LVEDP), which in turn is an approximation of left ventricular end-diastolic volume (LVEDV). These measurements enable the clinician to assess ventricular function and ventricular preload. The data derived from the pulmonary artery catheter can be misleading or misinterpreted due to airway pressure artifacts, abnormalities of cardiopulmonary function, and technical problems.

ETIOLOGY
I. Airway pressure artifacts
   A. Positive pressure
      1. Inspiratory phase with controlled ventilation
      2. Expiratory phase—active exhalation due to bronchospasm/chronic obstructive pulmonary disease (pursed lip breathing)
      3. Inspiratory/expiratory phases—continuous positive airway pressure
   B. Negative pressure artifacts—inspiratory phase of spontaneous ventilation
II. Abnormalities of cardiopulmonary function
   A. Congestive heart failure (CHF)
   B. Cardiac ischemia

C. Mitral stenosis/regurgitation
D. Ventricular septal defect
E. Low left atrial compliance
F. Atrioventricular dysynchrony
G. Adult respiratory distress syndrome
III. Technical problems
    A. "Permanent wedge"
    B. Transducer-related problems (see Chap. 55)

DISCUSSION

Estimation of left ventricular pressures from the pulmonary artery requires a continuous column of blood between the distal end of the pulmonary artery catheter and the ventricle. Placement of the catheter tip into a zone 3 lung unit will ensure this. Positional changes, drops in intravascular volume, or the addition of high positive end-expiratory pressure (PEEP) can transform zone 3 units to zone 2 or zone 1 (Fig. 54-1). When this occurs, positive and negative airway pressure artifacts can be transmitted to the pulmonary artery catheter depending on ventilatory mode, disease state, and severity of altered pulmonary or thoracic compliance.

To avoid incorporating the airway pressure artifacts into the PAOP measurements, the readings should be taken at end-expiration and interpreted from a paper printout. Recording PAOP from a digital display will result in erroneous data due to time averaging by the monitor. For patients with very rapid ventilatory rates or severe bronchospasm, measurement of airway pressures may be required. The measured artifact can then be subtracted from the PAOP. When using more than 10 cm H_2O pressure of PEEP, measurement of intrathoracic pressures may again be required. A less attractive alternative involves the measurement of PAOP during momentary cessation of PEEP once or twice daily to determine the amount of pressure that is transmitted. The latter will fluctuate with changes in compliance. PEEP of less than

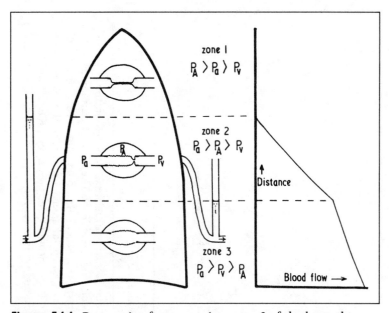

Figure 54-1. Progressing from zone 1 to zone 3 of the lung, the alveolar pressure (P_A) is seen to become less than the arterial (P_a) and venous (P_V) pressures. (From Benumof JL: Respiratory physiology and respiratory function during anesthesia. In Miller RD [ed]: *Anesthesia*, 2nd ed. New York: Churchill Livingstone, 1986.)

10 cm H_2O usually does not induce significant airway pressure artifact.

In the setting of interstitial lung disease and adult respiratory distress syndrome, elevations of pulmonary vascular resistance can lead to an underestimation of pulmonary capillary pressure (P_c) by PAOP. Various techniques are employed to estimate P_c using analyses of the PAOP waveform (Fig. 54-2). A current theory analysis of the waveform yields lower P_c estimations than the method used in Figure 54-2.

An understanding of the normal left atrial waveform as it relates to atrial and ventricular filling can be applied to the PAOP waveform to detect anomalies of physiology and anatomy (Fig. 54-3). Concurrent with atrial contraction there

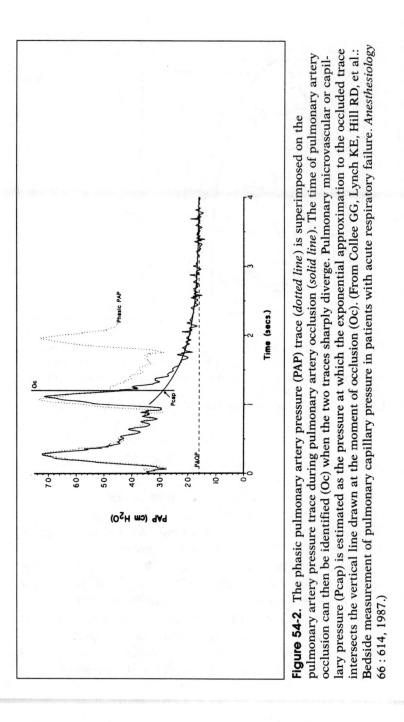

Figure 54-2. The phasic pulmonary artery pressure (PAP) trace (*dotted line*) is superimposed on the pulmonary artery pressure trace during pulmonary artery occlusion (*solid line*). The time of pulmonary artery occlusion can then be identified (Oc) when the two traces sharply diverge. Pulmonary microvascular or capillary pressure (Pcap) is estimated as the pressure at which the exponential approximation to the occluded trace intersects the vertical line drawn at the moment of occlusion (Oc). (From Collee GG, Lynch KE, Hill RD, et al.: Bedside measurement of pulmonary capillary pressure in patients with acute respiratory failure. *Anesthesiology* 66 : 614, 1987.)

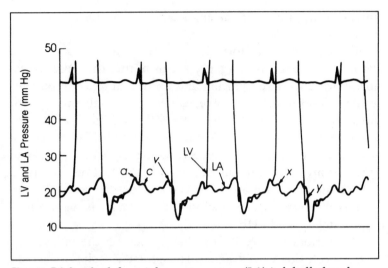

Figure 54-3. The left atrial pressure wave (LA) is labelled and superimposed with the left ventricular pressure wave (LV). a = a wave; c = c wave; v =v wave; x = x descent; y = y descent. (From Peterson KL, Ross J, Jr. : Cardiac catheterization and angiography. In Braunwald E, Isselbacher KJ, Petersdorf RG, [eds]: *Harrison's Principles of Internal Medicine*, 11th ed, New York : McGraw-Hill, 1987. P 892.)

is a positive deflection of the PAOP waveform known as the "a" wave. Left ventricular contraction ensues, causing descent of the cardiac base and bulging of the mitral valve into the left atrium, manifest as a second positive deflection denoted as the "c" wave. During ventricular systole, the atrium relaxes, causing a negative deflection wave defined as the "x" descent. As ventricular systole ends, passive filling of the atrium results in the "v" wave. It is followed by the "y" descent, representing the opening of the mitral valve.

Since the a and v waves represent clinically distinct anomalies, the identification of each wave is important. Simultaneous paper recordings of the electrocardiogram (ECG), the arterial waveform, and the pulmonary artery occlusion waveform are used. A vertical line drawn from the area of T wave of the ECG through the peak of the arterial waveform will intersect the pulmonary artery occlusion waveform near the v waves (Fig. 54-4).

Normal PAOP waveform is transmitted as a and v waves. Pathologic waves are larger and can mimic the PAOP waveform, preventing recognition and treatment of a "permanent wedge" condition. The a wave, by definition, only occurs with atrial contraction; that is, patients with atrial fibrillation cannot have a waves. Pathologic a waves occur with mitral stenosis, atrioventricular dysynchrony, and early CHF. Pathologic v waves are most often associated with mitral regurgitation where the normal c and v waves are fused together. Other causes of large v waves include mitral stenosis, ventricular septal defect, and CHF.

The normal a wave is not always seen on the pulmonary artery occlusion wave tracing. Thus, the PAOP should be read immediately prior to the arterial wave upstroke. Without the a wave, which occurs at the end of ventricular diastole, the LVEDP will be underestimated. Conversely, the etiology of large a waves can be explained by atrial contraction against a closed or stenotic mitral valve, which results in high pressures.

Mitral regurgitation, which occurs during ventricular systole, increases the size of the v wave (which represents passive filling of the atrium during systole). In the absence of a new murmur, the diagnosis of mitral regurgitation due to the appearance of a v wave is uncertain. This is explained by the pressure-volume relationship of the left atrium. If the atrium is compliant, or hypovolemic, or if the regurgitant volume is not excessive, then the v wave may not be impressive. Conversely, by decreasing the atrial compliance, the v wave can be increased (Fig. 54-4) without changing the amount of regurgitance. Aortic regurgitation can lead to an underestimation of LVEDP. During diastole, as regurgitant flow begins, it induces early closure of the mitral valve. Regurgitation continues, but the LVEDP is not transmitted due to closure of the valve. Another cause of an enlarged v wave is increased pulmonary venous flow. The etiology is a simple augmentation of the passive atrial filling v wave.

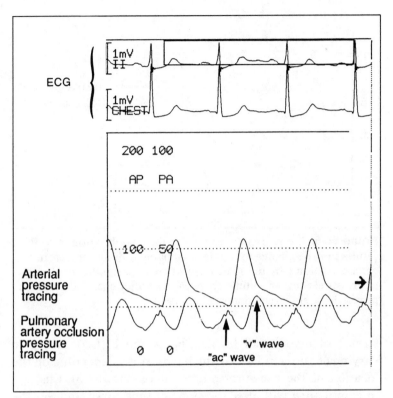

Figure 54-4. Timing of the arterial waveform and the pulmonary artery occlusion waveform, identifying a and v waves relative to the ECG complex.

Both a and v waves may occur during ischemia. The etiology of the a wave is the result of atrial contraction when ventricular compliance is decreased. As with mitral stenosis, there is a resistance to forward flow. The v wave can also signal ischemia when it is the result of acute papillary muscle dysfunction and subsequent mitral insufficiency.

The PAOP may not reflect left ventricular preload. A myriad of variables may preclude obtaining accurate left ventricular preload. The most careful measurements are merely reflective of LVEDP and not LVEDV, which better correlates to the

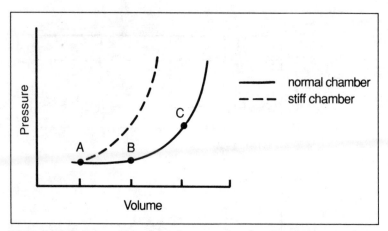

Figure 54-5. Increasing the volume in the chamber from A to B results in little change in pressure. Starting at B and increasing chamber volume by the same amount create a significant change in pressure. Similar volume changes in a stiffer chamber result in proportionately larger changes in pressure.

stretch of myocardial fibers. Changes in LVEDV will give varying changes in LVEDP during diastole, depending on the location of the pressure-volume curve (Fig. 54-5). Changes in compliance will alter the slope of that curve. Indeed, the PAOP can remain stable in the presence of ischemia and decreased ventricular filling. The value of the PAOP is best correlated with cardiac outputs and analysis of accompanying pulmonary artery occlusion waveform anomalies.

SELECTED READING

Mihm FG: Analysis of information pitfalls of pulmonary artery catheter monitoring. *ASA Refresher Courses Anesthesiol* 15 : 139, 1987.

Vender J: Pulmonary artery catharization and mixed venous oximetry: Update. *42nd Annual Refresher Course Lectures and Clinical Update Program.* American Society of Anesthesiologists. Lecture 265, pp 1–7.

55
Arterial Catheter

Theodore J. Heyneker

DEFINITION

There exists confusion among clinicians as to the significance
of what is measured using direct arterial pressure measurement, and how this correlates with indirect (blood pressure)
measurements. The interpretation of discrepancies between
the two techniques is likewise controversial. To add to this
chaos, improper calibrations and artifactual waveforms are
rampant.

External pressure transducers and their fluid-filled extension tubings used for direct blood pressure measurement
respond to the same physical laws that describe the motion of
a weight suspended by a spring. The fluid in the system has
mass, as does the suspended weight. The elasticity of the
extension tubing is analogous to the recoil of the spring. Oscillations in both systems are subject to frictional decay or
damping.

Every biologic system has a frequency response. For example, during audiometric testing, a determination of one's
aural frequency response is made. A noise stimulus above an
individual's frequency response will be neither heard nor
recorded. A pressure signal beyond the frequency range of an
arterial pressure transducing system will not be processed,
resulting in spuriously low blood pressure recordings. Analysis of arterial pressure waveforms reveals that they possess
significant energy at frequencies that are 5 to 10 times the
heart rate frequency. A heart rate of 60 beats/minute trans-
lates to one beat/second or 1 Hz. At this heart rate, a frequency

response of 5 to 10 Hz is required to ensure that the majority of pulse waveform energies are recorded.

The fluid-filled connecting tubing possesses its own natural frequency. When this frequency is attained, natural harmonics induce an augmentational distortion of the true waveform. Adding lengths of tubing decreases the natural or resonant frequency into the range of frequencies of the system presented by the arterial waveforms. This causes harmonic "ringing" or "overshoot," resulting in an overestimation of blood pressure. The resonant frequency of a particular transducer system can be measured by creating a square wave on the arterial waveform through a single rapid activation of the flushing mechanism. Using a paper trace at a fast speed, the resonant frequency is determined by dividing the paper speed (millimeters per second) by the millimeter distance between resulting resonant waveform peaks. If resonant frequency falls to 10 cycles/second, significant waveform overshoot of 20 to 30 percent may occur. If the connecting tubing in the system is very elastic, then energy and signal clarity are lost due to friction and an increased damping coefficient. Loss of high-frequency components results in an underestimation of pressure. Most systems have damping coefficients of 0.3 or less, which is roughly half the ideal damping coefficient.

Overall, a multitude of technical problems can lead to errors in arterial catheter waveforms.

ETIOLOGY

    I. Lack of calibration and balancing of the monitor
   II. Increased friction in the measuring system
      A. Kinked arterial catheter
      B. Blood clot on tip of the catheter
      C. Large air bubble in the connecting tubing
 III. Low natural frequencies (resonant frequencies)
      A. Long extension tubings/compliant extension tubing
      B. Small air bubbles
      C. Too many stopcocks

IV. Disappearance of waveform
   A. Monitor disconnect
   B. Blood pressure cuff inflation
   C. Malpositioned stopcock
   D. Monitor or calibration mode

DISCUSSION

Once optimal resonant frequency and damping coefficients are obtained, the system must be balanced and calibrated. Balancing the system requires electronic adjustment to reflect a "zero" pressure at heart level when the system is open to atmospheric pressure. An electronic signal can then be activated to verify a proper electronic calibration. Far too often this internal electronic test is deemed acceptable as a final calibration. True calibration requires testing of the transducer. By elevating the distal end of the fluid-filled pressure tubing system 67 cm above the recording transducer, a pressure of 50 mm Hg is generated. (Since mercury is 13.4 times heavier than water, a column of water 670 mm high is required to generate a pressure equal to that of a column of mercury 50 mm high.) By observing the corresponding electronic measurement, the relative accuracy of the transducer can be determined.

Most prepackaged transducer/tubing systems are created to have optimal resonant frequencies and damping coefficients. Yet even with proper calibration, accurate data are not obtained. The offending factors are inertia and friction of the fluid column connecting the patient to the transducer.

Increasing the friction of a system will dampen or flatten the pressure wave. Kinking of an arterial catheter, a blood clot on the tip of an arterial catheter, and a large air bubble in the tubing are potential etiologies. Incorrect calibration or gain settings on a monitor can cause the same effect, as can a partially loosened tubing to the stopcock connection. An acute change may also result from ipsilateral inflation of a blood pressure cuff. A gradual blunting of the pressure wave can be due to a transducer dome prepared and calibrated with excess contact fluid and a resultant high diaphragm pressure. Over time this pressure dissipates, causing the arterial waveform to fade. Total absence of a waveform may result from a loose or defective transducer, a malpositioned stopcock, or an amplifier that is still switched to calibration mode. All these factors should be considered *after* verifying the status of the patient.

Augmented or spiked waveforms are due to harmonic resonance. An ideal monitoring system possesses a natural frequency that is higher than the frequencies encountered in the pressure wave it measures. Though large catheters (18 gauge) help maintain higher natural frequencies, a smaller catheter is acceptable, since it has a higher damping coefficient, which mitigates overshoot. Long extension tubings lower the natural frequency of a system, enhancing the potential for a "ringing" effect. Stopcocks create the same effect due to their narrow internal diameter. Small air bubbles increase movement of the fluid in the system, thereby decreasing the natural frequency response. This effect is mimicked by using more compliant connecting tubing. By employing a system with a lowered frequency response, the potential exists for "overshoot" in peak pressure measurements; that is, blood pressure readings will be inaccurately elevated. This overshoot will vary over time with heart rate. Since the frequency of a rapid heart rate is higher, it more closely approximates the natural frequency of a system, potentially resulting in overshoot, whereas a decrease in heart rate lowers the heart rate frequency, thereby preventing overshoot.

SELECTED READING

Gravenstein JS, Paulus DA: *Clinical Monitoring Practice*, 2nd ed. Philadelphia: Lippincott, 1987. Pp 70–101.
Miller RD: *Anesthesia*, 3rd ed. New York: Churchill Livingstone, 1990. Pp 1035–1043.

56
Capnography

Theodore J. Heyneker

DEFINITION

Capnography refers to the curvilinear representation of the concentration of exhaled (and sometimes inhaled) carbon dioxide as a function of time. With ongoing ventilation one can easily discern a phasic pattern of the capnograph with inhalation or exhalation. Analysis of the resultant curves can be made in much the same fashion as one would analyze the various phases of an action potential.

The normal capnograph waveform comprises four phases:

Phase I is the baseline, which should be essentially zero (0.3 mm Hg) when additional carbon dioxide has not been added to the inspiratory gases. This phase represents the end of inspiration, inspiratory pause, and the clearing of dead space gas during the onset of expiration (Fig. 56-1).

Phase II shows a rapid increase in carbon dioxide concentration. This reflects the initial expiration of alveolar gases.

Phase III is the plateau phase, representing true alveolar carbon dioxide concentration. Due to variations in alveolar emptying times, this portion of the capnograph is never truly horizontal.

Phase IV represents the onset of inspiration. The point of intersection with phase I of the subsequent breath does not necessarily reflect the cessation of inspiration. It merely reflects the point at which the nadir of carbon dioxide tension is first attained.

Carbon dioxide can be measured using infrared devices or mass spectrometry. The derived data from either method are

283

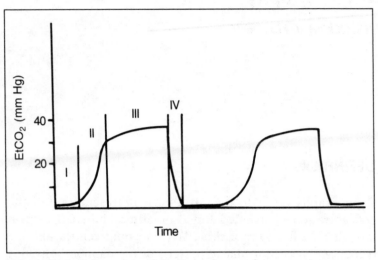

Figure 56-1. Delineation of the four phases of a capnogram. $EtCO_2$ = end-tidal carbon dioxide.

presented in the same fashion. Any capnograph, if used simply as a capnometer (that is, to read only the highest carbon dioxide concentration), may result in misinformation as well as a loss of information. Assessment of the capnogram itself will attest to the relative reliability of the data available or give clues as to the cause of the error, since anomalies can occur in all four phases.

ETIOLOGY
  I. Anomalies of phase I
    A. Addition of carbon dioxide to the fresh gas flow
    B. Bypassing the circle system carbon dioxide absorber
    C. Mispacking of the carbon dioxide absorber of a circle system (channeling)
    D. Expiratory valve incompetence
    E. Low fresh gas flow in a valveless breathing system
 II. Anomalies of phase II
    A. Variable alveolar emptying times

    B. Prolonged expiratory phase due to chronic obstructive pulmonary disease/bronchospasm

    C. Kinked endotracheal tube

III. Anomalies of phase III

    A. Anomalies of phase II

    B. Attempts at spontaneous ventilation

    C. Pushing and tugging by the surgeon

    D. Cardiac ejections

    E. Tachypnea

    F. Increased dead space

    G. Administration of sodium bicarbonate

IV. Anomalies of phase IV

    A. Slow sampling rates

    B. Low inspiratory gas flow rates

    C. Water trap

 V. Other

    A. Different gas flow in sampling line

    B. Water vapor pressure

    C. Pulmonary embolus

    D. Nonventilation

    E. Cardiac arrest

    F. Malignant hyperthermia

    G. Esophageal intubation

DISCUSSION

In phase I, if the baseline fails to return to zero, then carbon dioxide rebreathing is occurring. Possible etiologies include the addition of carbon dioxide to inspired gases, a circle system carbon dioxide absorber that is bypassed, spent, or mispacked, circle system expiratory valve incompetence, and the use of a valveless breathing circuit, such as the Maplesons, where rebreathing is inversely proportional to fresh gas flow. Using specially adapted nasal prongs or oxygen masks that allow gas sampling in well-draped patients undergoing ophthalmologic procedures, one may detect a degree of carbon dioxide rebreathing. This may be ameliorated by increasing oxygen flows and by partial lifting of the drapes. In these cases, the phase III carbon dioxide concentration will be inaccurate, but useful information can be obtained through trend analysis and observance of ventilatory rate.

If the slope of phase II is decreased, then by definition the rate of rise of carbon dioxide concentration in the expired gas is slowed. This slowing can be caused by variations in alveolar emptying times, or it can be a reflection of the prolonged expiratory phase of chronic obstructive pulmonary disease (COPD) or bronchospasm. Mechanically induced expiratory flow retardation such as a kinked or partially clogged endotracheal tube can also present in this manner.

A normal phase III should tend toward the horizontal. Increases in slope in phase III are a result of a retardation of expiratory flow, with the same differential diagnosis as noted for decreases in the slope of phase II. Irregularly spaced dips in the plateau of phase III may be attributed to attempts at spontaneous ventilation in the mechanically ventilated patient. Consideration should be given as to the possible etiologies of air hunger. Hiccoughs can present in a similar fashion.

Another cause for phase III irregularities can be the pushing or pulling of the surgeon on the abdomen or chest. In this case, pushing by the surgeon may present as an upward deflection on the plateau as carbon dioxide is forced out of the lungs. Pulling by the surgeon may induce negative intrathoracic pressure and the entrainment of fresh gas, momentarily diminishing the carbon dioxide concentration at the sampling unit.

Regularly placed phase III variations of a sinusoidal pattern may correlate in frequency with the heart rate. Normal cardiac ejections can change intrathoracic volume enough to generate inspiratory, then expiratory gas flow. These cardiac-induced gas flows can sometimes be measured using in-circuit respirometry on mechanically ventilated patients.

The definition of phase III refers to a "plateau phase." Degeneration from a box-like capnogram to a rounded shape can best be seen in rapid shallow breathing, such as might occur in a pediatric patient during mask induction. In these patients, the dead space of the mask limits most, if not all, carbon dioxide from reaching the sampling port. A unique aberration of the phase III plateau (Fig. 56-2) was attributed to a loose Luer-lock connection in the sampling line, resulting in the entrainment of room air and a lower-than-normal carbon dioxide plateau concentration. At the onset of each positive-pressure inspiration, the pressure gradient across the sampling line causes increased end-expiratory gas flow in the sampling line and therefore less entrainment of room air. The highest carbon dioxide concentration on this unusual capnogram was very close to that measured when the loose connection was tightened.

When the slope of phase IV becomes less vertical, several etiologies must be considered: slow sampling rates, very low inspiratory gas flow rates, and partial rebreathing. In contrast, a peak in the carbon dioxide level in phase IV that is airway pressure dependent has been recorded. High airway pressures compress gas in the water trap; some gas collects at the bottom of the trap, along with humidity. The carbon dioxide concentration at the bottom of the trap is an average of previous samplings. This gas expands when the peak pressure decreases during expiration (i.e., phase III, early phase IV). It then remixes with gas in the sampling catheter, and this abnormal mixture is reflected on the capnograph. The artifact appears out of phase with the ventilatory cycle (i.e., it seems to occur during inspiration) because the errant sample does not have to travel the distance of the sampling tubing. Reducing the size of the water trap causes the artifact to disappear (Fig. 56-3).

Problems can arise that are not unique to any particular phase of the expiration waveform. Long gas-sampling lines for mass spectrometry can result in inaccurate data, a situation aggravated by ventilatory rates greater than 50 times/minute. Differential resistance to gas flow and dissolution of carbon dioxide into the sampling catheter can result in near

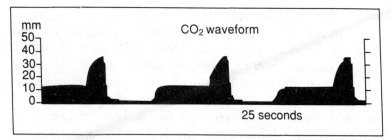

Figure 56-2. Abnormal capnogram caused by a loose sampling port connection. This can be recreated by loosening the connection at the water trap. (Modified from Martin M, Zupan J: Unusual end-tidal CO_2 waveform. *Anesthesiology* 66 : 712, 1987.)

normal waveforms, with inaccurately low carbon dioxide concentrations; it can also present with distortions consistent with COPD. The catheter use for remote mass spectrometric sampling is made of either polyethylene, polyvinylchloride, nylon, or Teflon. Mass spectrometers with nylon catheters are less likely to manifest distortion. The frequency response and accuracy of long sampling catheters can be improved with minor adjustments in the electronic circuit.

The preceding paragraph refers to differential resistance of gas flow in long mass spectrometry sampling lines. This causes certain gas molecules to flow faster than others, resulting in a mixing of gases. It can also occur in infrared carbon dioxide analyzers at ventilatory rates in excess of 31 times/minute. The issue can be resolved by using an in-line analyzer, but cost, dead space, and weight sometimes render this impractical.

Another potential problem in accuracy exists with several infrared carbon dioxide analyzers. Sampling catheter material used on these monitors effectively removes water vapor prior to gas analysis. This has led to a calibration by some manufacturers that disregards the 47 mm Hg of water vapor that exists at 37°C. The result is a carbon dioxide reading 6.6 percent higher than exists in the patient.

Slow changes in peak carbon dioxide concentrations as recorded by the capnograph are rarely alarming, since they

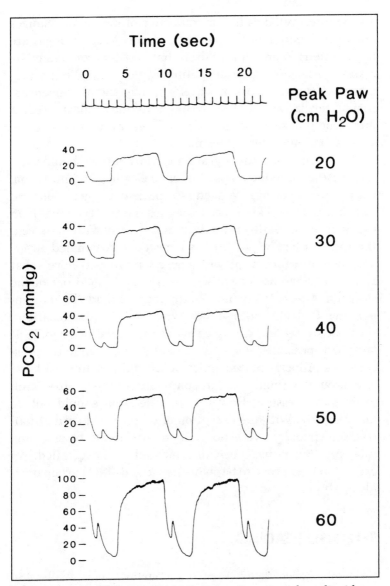

Figure 56-3. Peak airway-dependent inspiratory carbon dioxide peaks. (From van Genderingen HR, Gravenstein N: Capnogram artifact during high airway pressures caused by a water trap. *Anesth. Analg.* 66 : 181, 1987.)

can be interpreted as merely reflective of metabolic changes due to the cooling of the patient or fever. Acute changes are more serious. A precipitous drop that is still accompanied by a waveform may represent pulmonary embolization; a precipitous drop with loss of waveform may signal nonventilation or cardiac arrest. A fast-rising level may reflect a recent intravenous dose of sodium bicarbonate, or it may be an early sign of malignant hyperthermia.

The absence of a capnogram after intubation should alert the anesthetist to the possibility of an esophageal intubation. Only after ascertaining adequate patient oxygenation and ventilation should alternative diagnoses be entertained. If an esophageal intubation is made after difficulty with mask ventilation or after the patient has ingested a carbonated beverage, then the capnograph will show a series of waveforms that stair-step down as the carbon dioxide is washed out of the stomach. Alternatively, no reading may be made by the capnometer. If all clinical signs point to a well-ventilated patient, then one might tentatively consider the capnometer to be at fault. One possible cause of an absent capnogram in the presence of a properly placed endotracheal tube is due to a large leak around a small tube, in conjunction with positive end-expiratory pressure. However, this decision should not be taken lightly. With the exception of direct vocal cord visualization, virtually every noncapnometric mode of assessing tube placement has been documented to have failed. An exception may prove to be colorimetric end-tidal carbon dioxide analysis.

SELECTED READING

Good ML: Capnography: Uses, interpretations and pitfalls. *ASA Refresher Course Anesthesiol* 18 : 175, 1990.
Raemer DB, Francis D, Philip JH, Gabel RA: Variation in P_{CO_2} between arterial blood and peak expired gas during anesthesia. *Anesth Analg* 62 : 1, 1983.

57
Changes in Electroencephalogram

Theodore J. Heyneker

DEFINITION

The electroencephalogram (EEG) is a continuous recording of spontaneous cortical electrical activity. These electrical signals reflect excitatory and inhibitory postsynaptic potentials generated by cortical pyramidal cells and their dendritic trees. The resulting waveforms are analyzed according to frequency, amplitude, and symmetry. The resulting data can be used to monitor the cerebral cortex.

There are four frequency classifications. High-frequency rhythms (13–30 Hz), referred to as beta activity, are usually reflective of mental concentration in the awake subject. Slightly slower frequencies (8–13 Hz) are termed alpha waves and reflect relaxed alertness with the eyes closed. Theta rhythms (4–8 Hz) are commonly seen during sleep or with anesthesia in adults; they are also frequently seen in normal, awake, hyperventilated children. Delta waves (0–4 Hz) are seen with deep sleep or deep anesthesia, or they can be indicative of brain tumors.

EEG patterns are affected by many factors, which include the depth of anesthesia, arterial blood pressure, arterial blood gas tensions, hematocrit, patient position, body temperature, and the intensity of stimulation. Controlling or minimizing changes induced by these variables is necessary if changes due to ischemia or hypoxia are to be detected.

ETIOLOGY

I. Depth of anesthesia
    A. Inhalational anesthetics

    B. Barbiturates
    C. Opioids
    D. Ketamine
    E. Benzodiazepines
II. Physiologic changes
    A. Hypoxemia
    B. Hypoperfusion
    C. Hypocarbia
    D. Temperature
III. Other
    A. Space-occupying lesions
    B. Trauma
    C. Intensity of stimulation

DISCUSSION

As a general rule, an increase in anesthetic depth will induce a progression from high frequency to slower frequencies. This will continue to evolve toward periods of suppression with intermittent bursts of activity indicative of incomplete central nervous system suppression. Ultimately, electrical quiescence ensues. For volatile anesthetics at concentrations of less than 1 MAC there is a predominance of beta activity. As the depth of anesthesia increases with halothane, there is a shift to theta and delta waves, ending with suppression at 2 MAC. Increasing inspired enflurane concentration can cause spike and wave patterns; seizure activity may be precipitated by auditory stimulation when such patterns are present. Isoflurane is more like halothane than enflurane, producing slower waveforms with increased anesthetic dose. Isoflurane progresses more rapidly to burst suppression than halothane and more readily induces electrical silence. Hypercapnia generally has an additive effect on EEG suppression. Hypocapnia lowers the seizure threshold when using enflurane. Spikes without seizures can occur when hypocapnia and isoflurane are used together. The effects of nitrous oxide on the EEG show a parallel decrease in frequency as the concentration of the gas is increased, although high-frequency components may occur.

Barbiturates demonstrate a dose-dependent slowing of frequency, beginning with a pattern of fast activity when slow infusions are administered. Faster drug administration attenuates the high-frequency phase, resulting in rapid progression to delta activity, at which time surgical incision is tolerated. Continued drug administration will result in an isoelectric EEG. Etomidate behaves in much the same manner as the barbiturates, although it may activate epileptogenic sites, thus precluding its use in patients with seizure disorders. Propofol rapidly produces delta-wave activity, but unlike barbiturates, the slow-frequency waves are accompanied by spindle activity in the 11 to 13 Hz range. Benzodiazepines effect a dose-dependent slowing of EEG frequency with an accompanying rise in seizure threshold. Ketamine stimulates high-frequency EEG patterns (30–40 Hz), which correlate well with its ability to produce hallucinations and subcortical seizure activity. Higher doses can subsequently proceed to theta- and delta-wave patterns. Droperidol, which is also a dissociative drug, produces remarkably little EEG effect.

Anesthetic induction with opioids shows initial diminution of alpha and beta activity occurring within minutes before progressing to delta activity. Without redosing, a regression to faster frequencies will occur. Extremely high doses do not result in EEG quiescence; in fact, high-dose narcotic administration has produced EEG seizure activity in animals. Seizure activity has been reported with lower doses of fentanyl, but these cases are without EEG corroboration. Normeperidine, a metabolite of meperidine, is a cerebral irritant and possibly epileptogenic.

Changes in various physiologic parameters correlate with the deterioration of normal EEG patterns to slower frequencies and ultimately to flat EEGs. As can be seen in Figure 57-1, a severe degree of arterial hypoxemia is required to effect a slowing of the EEG and loss of consciousness. The initial slowing of the EEG does not occur until the saturation of a

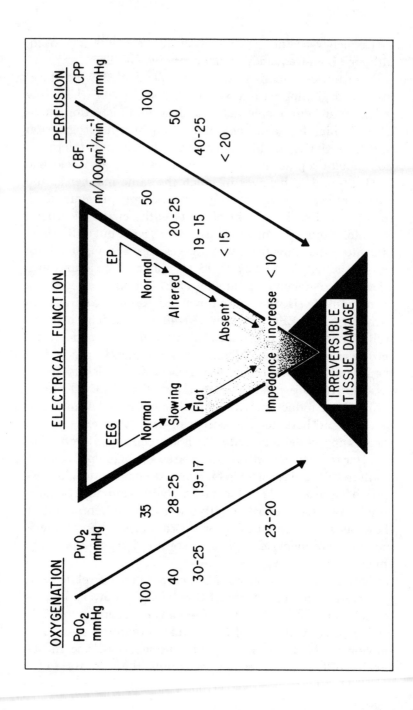

relatively normal hemoglobin concentration falls below 70 percent. Hypocarbia can increase EEG amplitude while slowing rhythms to the delta-theta range. These effects are minimized with an increase in arterial oxygen content and with nitrates, indicating that the induced EEG changes are due to vasoconstriction. Hypercarbia results in beta-wave activity until carbon dioxide levels near 200 mm Hg are reached, at which time EEG slowing occurs.

Arterial blood pressure and the effects of patient positioning can also alter the EEG indirectly through effects on cerebral blood flow (CBF) and cerebral perfusion pressure (CPP). It can be discerned from Figure 57-1 that decreases in CBF to 40 percent of normal will induce a significant slowing, if not a flattening, of the EEG pattern. Decreases in CPP of similar proportions effect the same significant slowing of EEG frequency.

Space-occupying lesions in the brain are not electrically active. Changes in EEG due to tumors are most likely due to lack of electrical activity as well as to alterations in blood flow to areas surrounding the tumor. Infratentorial tumors can induce slow-frequency rhythms that are symmetric across the midsagittal line due to displacement of the centrencephalon. Cortical tumors can present with very slow unilateral or bilateral EEG rhythms that are a function of the tumor location. As a result of swelling or impedance to vascular flow, delta waves should not be unexpected. The amplitude of the EEG might be decreased locally due to space-occupying tumors, abscesses, or hematoma due to the increased distance from the pyramidal cells to the skin surface.

Figure 57-1. Arterial hypoxemia is associated with slowing of the electroencephalogram (EEG). EP = evoked potentials; CBF = cerebral blood flow; CPP = cerebral perfusion pressure. (From Shapiro HM: Anesthesia effects upon cerebral blood flow, cerebral metabolism, electroencephalogram, and evoked potentials [and] neurosurgical anesthesia and intracranial hypertension. In Miller RD [ed]: *Anesthesia*, 2nd ed. New York: Churchill Livingstone, 1986.)

Cerebral trauma results in decreases in EEG amplitude and EEG slowing. Mild injuries are self-limiting, but more severe injuries progress to delta-wave activity (0–4 Hz) with attendant poor prognoses. Recovery, if it occurs, requires several months for normalization of the EEG. Post-traumatic epileptogenic spike can occur from localized trauma.

EEG monitoring is used most frequently in the operating room for carotid endarterectomies under general anesthesia, for patients undergoing cardiopulmonary bypass, and during the use of induced hypotension. During carotid endarterectomy, EEG changes will not occur unless significant changes in CBF occur on the affected side. The existence of a complete circle of Willis may preclude such changes. If symptomatic EEG changes do occur, they present as diffuse ipsilateral slowing with loss of amplitude, both of which are consistent with hypoperfusion and hypoxia. Such changes are more readily detected by EEG than by somatosensory evoked potentials. If an infarct occurs, it will present as localized areas of delta-wave activity several hours after the insult. Focal lesions are less likely to produce loss of consciousness. EEG changes of less than 10 minutes' duration do not usually correlate with postoperative deficits.

To use intraoperative EEG monitoring effectively, one must separate anesthetic-induced EEG changes from those changes resulting from physiologic aberrations. It is imperative that anesthetic techniques be chosen to minimize pharmacologic effects on the EEG, thus retaining some degree of electrical activity. Those physiologic variables affecting the EEG that are under the control of the anesthesiologist should also be manipulated to minimize these effects on the EEG. Pharmacologic and physiologic variables should then be maintained, where possible, at a steady state to allow a baseline EEG activity against which any unexpected changes can be compared. These conditions will enable the diagnosis of ischemia and the institution of appropriate therapies to begin promptly.

SELECTED READING

Cucchiara RF, Michenfelder JD: *Clinical Neuroanesthesia.* New York: Churchill Livingstone, 1990. Pp 118–139.

Levy WJ: Intraoperative EEG patterns: Implications for EEG monitoring. *Anesthesiology* 60 : 430, 1984.

58
Changes in Somatosensory Evoked Potentials

Theodore J. Heyneker

DEFINITION

A newly developed neurologic monitor is the evoked potential (EP). It is a graphic representation of the electrophysiologic responses of the nervous system to, in most cases, sensory stimuli. There are three subsets of sensory evoked potentials (SEP) classified according to the type of stimulation used: (1) visual evoked potentials (VEP), which are used during surgery proximal to the optic nerve; (2) brainstem auditory evoked potentials (BAEP), which are used during posterior cranial fossa surgery; and (3) somatosensory evoked potentials (SSEP), which are used primarily during spinal and spinal cord surgery. Since SEPs generate low-amplitude signals when compared to nonevoked electroencephalogram (EEG) recordings, they require amplification and summation of repetitive time-locked stimulation. The result is graphed as a function of time (stimulus to waveform latencies) and voltage (waveform amplitudes).

The SSEP waveforms are categorized as belonging to either far field or near field. Far-field potentials arise in peripheral nerves, the spinal cord, or subcortical brain structures using brain tissue as a conductive medium to travel quickly to the scalp recording sites, resulting in short latencies due to the speed of conduction. Low-voltage amplitudes also occur due to dissipation of energy in brain tissue through which the impulse has travelled. The near-field potential travels through multiple brain synapses and is processed by them, resulting in longer latencies. Its last electrical potential is created near the recording scalp electrode (or it can be recorded at the spinal cord near the site of impulse generation).

Monitoring SSEPs, by definition, can only detect deficits in the dorsal column. This limitation is balanced by the capability of monitoring the entire neuraxis. The posterior tibial nerve at the ankle and the median nerves at the wrist are the most common sites of stimulation for SSEP recording. Posterior tibial nerve responses can be recorded at the popliteal fossa, lumbar, thoracic, and contralateral cortical sites. Median nerve responses are recorded at Erb's point (lateral neck at C6), C7, C2, and the contralateral somatosensory cortex. A useful application of this technique compares upper and lower extremity SSEPs to detect potential spinal cord injury due to ischemia or infarction during thoracic aortic surgery. For unilateral tumor or structural lesions, especially above C7, the contralateral SSEP is used as the control. SSEPs are also used to assess demyelination and brain death.

Describing SSEP waveform morphology is confusing because of nonstandardized nomenclature and variation in sites of stimulation for the distal median nerve. It is accepted that the first near-field deflection has a latency of 15 to 20 msec. Subsequent deflections of the same polarity are referred to as N waves, numbered N_1, N_2, $N_3 \rightarrow N_\infty$. The waveform pattern is classically described as a "V" or "W". Interspersed deflections of the opposite polarity are connoted P_1, P_2, P_3, and so forth. When citing specific examples, the waveforms are described by their actual latencies (e.g., N_{20}, P_{22}) (Fig. 58-1). Whether N

Figure 58-1. The waveforms are labeled "P" or "N" according to institutional convention. The numerical subscripts indicate post-stimulus latency. The waveform on the left is derived from median nerve stimulation at the wrist. The waveform on the right results from posterior tibial nerve stimulation at the ankle. (From Grundy BL: Intraoperative monitoring of sensory-evoked potentials. *Anesthesiology* 58 : 72, 1983.)

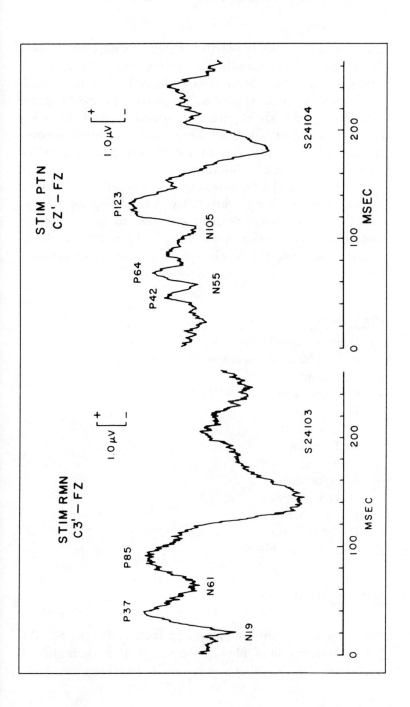

deflections are actually positive or negative depends on how the polarity of the recording electrodes is arranged. Waveforms preceding the initial near-field deflection are recording from Erb's point (P_9) or at the proximal cervical spinal cord (N_{13}). There are significant variabilities in latency between subjects, but since each subject serves as his or her own control, this is not of concern for individual patient management. Baseline SSEPs should be obtained preoperatively to determine optimal stimulation sites and baseline waveforms for such control. Due to variability in recording techniques, each laboratory should determine its own ranges for normal amplitudes and latency. Alterations in the SSEP from baseline are due to anesthesia, physiologic changes, and technical problems.

ETIOLOGY

  I. Depth of anesthesia
    A. Inhalational anesthetics
    B. Opioids
    C. Barbiturates
    D. Ketamine
    E. Etomidate
    F. Propofol
 II. Physiologic changes
    A. Hypoxemia
    B. Hypercapnia
    C. Hypoperfusion
    D. Temperature
III. Technical problems

DISCUSSION

The most significant nonpathologic factor affecting SSEP is the administration of inhalational anesthetics. Their effect is dose-dependent, causing a decrease in waveform amplitude and an increase in latency. Waveforms are almost totally lost at 1.0 to 1.5 MAC. The effects are most pronounced with enflurane and least with halothane (Fig. 58-2). The addition of 60% nitrous oxide further diminishes waveform amplitude and increases latency.

Intravenous anesthetics, like inhalational anesthetics, can affect SSEPs in a dose-related fashion but not to the same degree. Low doses of morphine and fentanyl can produce increases in latency with variable changes in amplitude. Thiopental at high dosages can significantly decrease amplitude and increase latency but not to the point of precluding the use of SSEPs as a monitor. Etomidate, propofol, and ketamine have been shown to increase amplitude. These changes must merely be taken into account when diagnosing potentially pathologic waveforms. Noncortical evoked responses are much less sensitive to the effects of anesthetic agents.

Hypothermia can affect SSEPs. With mild hypothermia (35–36°C) the effect is minimal. In the range of 27 to 35°C, there occurs a linear increase in latency of 1 msec/°C. At temperatures as low as 18°C, SSEPs can still be recorded, but the increase in latency becomes exponential relative to the temperature decline. Local cooling through use of irrigation and intravenous fluids can also affect SSEPs. Conversely, at high temperatures (41–42°C), there is an absence of detectable SSEP.

Both blood gas tensions and blood pressure can affect SSEP waveform. Hypercapnia and hypoxemia may induce deleterious effects. Hypocapnia as measured by end-tidal carbon dioxide tension to levels of 20 mm Hg does not significantly affect SSEPs. Hypotension and lack of perfusion can have a significant impact on SSEP; with induction of deliberate hypotension, a reassessment of "baseline" SSEPs is required prior to beginning surgical manipulations that may induce changes.

This type of monitoring can be fraught with technical problems simply due to the multiple electrical contacts required. Elevated impedance at the recording electrode is most

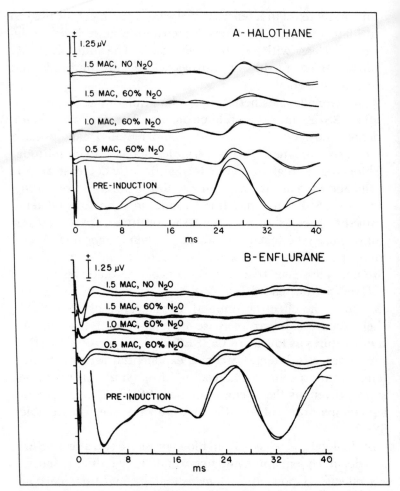

Figure 58-2. The effect of inhaled anesthetics on cortical evoked potentials. (From Peterson DO, Drummond JC, Todd MM: Effects of halothane, enflurane, isoflurane, and nitrous oxide on somatosensory evoked potentials in humans. *Anesthesiology* 65 : 39, 1986.)

frequently a problem. Failure to deliver an appropriate stimulus due to lack of electrode contact is another. Electrical and mechanical noise in the area can alter the signals (e.g., "bovie" interference).

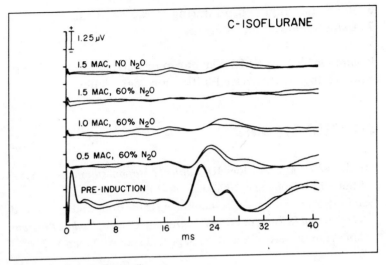

Figure 58-2 (continued).

There are no specific definitions as to what constitutes a significant change in SSEP relative to predicting outcomes. It is generally accepted that the degree of waveform change is proportional to outcome. A reasonable guideline for what constitutes a "significant" change would be a reduction in amplitude of greater than 50 percent and an increase in latency of 10 percent. Loss of waveform, however, is generally accepted as significant. Return of waveform to normal in the recovery room has been associated with good outcome. When "significant" waveform changes are present or when loss of waveform occurs, institution of the following interventions should be considered:

1. Increasing oxygen tension
2. Increasing hematocrit
3. Increasing blood pressure
4. Removing or repositioning retractors
5. Lessening tension on spinal curvature for associated surgery

6. Repositioning the head during intracranial surgery
7. Using mannitol and steroids

Permanent loss of SSEP waveform or persistence of "significant" change is associated with neurologic deficit.

SELECTED READING

Cucchiara RF, Michenfelder JD: *Clinical Neuroanesthesia.* New York: Churchill Livingstone, 1990. Pp 139–149.
Mahla M: Electrophysiologic monitoring of the brain and spinal cord. *41st Annual Refresher Course Lectures and Clinical Update Program.* American Society of Anesthesiologists. Lecture 522, pp 1–7.

59
Automatic Blood Pressure Cuffs

Theodore J. Heyneker

DEFINITION

Automatic blood pressure measuring devices use the Doppler method, auscultation, and oscillometric techniques. The Arteriosonde (Roche Medical, Cranburg, NJ) employs a Doppler signal. It uses a motion detector to identify the onset of arterial wall motion caused by the resumption of blood flow as the pressure in the occluding cuff is decreased. The Infrasond (Puritan-Bennett, Los Angeles, CA) uses microphones to auscultate Korotkoff sounds; that is, it uses the Riva-Rocci method. More familiar to the operating room setting is the Dinamap (Critikon Medical, Tampa, FL), which measures the onset and cessation of arterial pulse wave pressure oscillations and their amplitudes as the measured pressure of the cuff diminishes. This discussion will focus on problems that may be encountered using the Dinamap.

ETIOLOGY
I. Patient-related problems
   A. Voluntary movement
   B. Fasciculations
   C. Seizures
   D. Irregular heart rhythms
   E. Bradycardia

II. Technical problems
   A. Cuff size
   B. Monitor calibration
   C. Hose leaks

DISCUSSION

To determine systolic blood pressure, the Dinamap inflates the cuff pressure to a preset level of 178 mm Hg for adults. A high-amplitude oscillation detected at this point induces a further increase in cuff pressure. Once the desired low-amplitude or absent oscillations are detected, a stepped pressure deflation occurs. The pressure is diminished each time two oscillations or pulsations of equal amplitude are detected or every 1.6 seconds, whichever comes first. This sequence is repeated until oscillation amplitude diminishes significantly, indicating the diastolic pressure (or until the cuff pressure drops below 7 mm Hg). The mean arterial pressure (MAP) is determined from the cuff pressure measured when oscillation amplitude is maximal.

Detection of the first and last oscillations is required to determine systolic and diastolic blood pressures. The thresholds for oscillation detection may match oscillations due to fine muscular tremors and thereby result in low diastolic blood pressure readings. Patient movement at any time may cause a misreading of MAP; a surgeon leaning on a cuff may produce the same effect. Convulsions or unrestrained patient movement may preclude blood pressure measurement.

Regardless of the method used for indirect blood pressure measurement, an improperly sized cuff will induce measurement error. A small cuff will falsely elevate blood pressure. A loose cuff may result in no readings, or it may falsely elevate the readings. A large cuff will falsely lower blood pressure.

Monthly calibration measurements can detect small cuff and connecting hose leaks, which may otherwise not be detected. These leaks may cause a more rapid step deflation of the cuff and result in a falsely low blood pressure. Alternatively, the leaks may not be detected until they are large enough to preclude maintenance of a given cuff pressure long enough to measure the amplitudes of two oscillations. In this case, the automatic blood pressure measurement device will simply fail to produce a reading.

Irregular cardiac rhythms can confound these machines. Recall that the monitor is trying to detect two oscillations of equal amplitude at any given pressure step. Variations of left ventricular ejection due to irregular left ventricular filling times may extend the search time for "paired oscillations," thereby prolonging the time required to determine a blood pressure. Irregular pauses in left ventricular injection for more than 1.6 seconds may cause the monitor to decrease cuff pressure to the "next step." Should this happen at points coinciding with systolic or diastolic blood pressures, erroneous data may be presented. In addition, bradycardias will confuse the monitor. The stepwise degradation in cuff pressure will occur every 1.6 seconds if "paired" oscillations are not detected. A simple mathematical exercise will explain the lack of displayed readings at heart rates of less than 38 beats/minute.

The lack of correlation between invasive and noninvasive blood pressure measurements is well documented. The most significant differences occur with hypertension, hypotension, hypothermia, and obesity. Comparisons of Riva-Rocci and intra-arterial systolic and diastolic pressure show good correlation only when the pressure measured intra-arterially was obtained in the same manner Korotkoff sounds are obtained (i.e., as flow returned after cuff occlusion). This illustrates that the intra-arterial catheter measures *pressure* directly, while the cuff measurements gauge *flow* directly and attempt indirectly to measure pressure.

This does not mean that indirect pressure measurements are inaccurate. The opposite could be argued, citing indirect measurements as the historical gold standard. In stable patients with concurrent pulse oximetry and end-tidal carbon dioxide measurement, the use of an automatic blood pressure measuring device can be an acceptable alternative to the cost and potential morbidity of direct blood pressure measurements.

SELECTED READING

Barash PG, Cullen BF, Stoelting RK: *Clinical Anesthesia.* Philadelphia: Lippincott, 1989. Pp 566–567.
Gravenstein JS, Paulus DA: *Clinical Monitoring Practice.* 2nd ed. Philadelphia: Lippincott, 1987. Pp 50–70.

IX
Obstetrics

60
Changes in Fetal Heart Tracings

DEFINITION

The fetal heart tracing, a graphic display of the fetal heart rate (FHR), consists of three components. The first is beat-to-beat variability, a term referring to the fluctuation of 3 to 8 beats/minute that characterizes a normal fetal heart tracing. The second component is the rate of the fetal heartbeat. The third is decelerations (or decels), which occur transiently and are categorized according to their temporal relationship to the uterine contractions. Some changes in the fetal heart tracings may be benign, while others indicate fetal compromise. These changes fall into four major categories: (1) decreased beat-to-beat variability, (2) sinus tachycardia, (3) sinus bradycardia, and (4) decelerations (early, variable, and late).

ETIOLOGY

I. Decreased beat-to-beat variability
   A. Fetal hypoxia
   B. Fetal sleep states
   C. Central nervous system (CNS) depressant drugs (narcotics)
   D. Parasympatholytics (atropine, scopolamine)
   E. Cardiac abnormalities
   F. CNS abnormalities (anencephaly)
   G. Prematurity
II. Sinus tachycardia (heart rate > 160 beats/minute)
   A. Fetal hypoxia
   B. Fetal infection (amnionitis)
   C. Anemia

D. Maternal fever
E. Maternal drug use (cocaine)
III. Sinus bradycardia (heart rate < 120 beats/minute)
   A. Fetal hypoxia
   B. Umbilical cord compression
   C. Head compression
   D. Postparacervical block
IV. Decelerations
   A. Early: head compression
   B. Variable
      1. Umbilical cord compression
      2. Mild hypoxia
   C. Late: uteroplacental insufficiency
      1. Vascular abnormalities (preeclampsia, diabetes mellitus)
      2. Uterine hyperstimulation (oxytocin)
      3. Maternal hypotension (regional anesthesia, aorto-caval compression)
      4. Severe myocardial hypoxia

DISCUSSION

The early detection of abnormalities in the fetal heart tracing and correction of the causes of these abnormalities are important to overall fetal outcome. When a change in the FHR pattern is detected, the first and foremost intervention is to ensure adequate fetal oxygenation; administering supplemental oxygen to the mother and ensuring left lateral uterine displacement may avert fetal hypoxia.

Beat-to-beat variability represents the normal interaction between the fetal sympathetic and parasympathetic nervous systems and the fetal cardiac conduction system (Fig. 60-1). It is an important indicator of adequate oxygenation of the fetal heart and CNS. Early stages of fetal hypoxia lead to disruption in the integrity of the normal physiologic pathways and loss of beat-to-beat variability. Nonasphyxia causes of

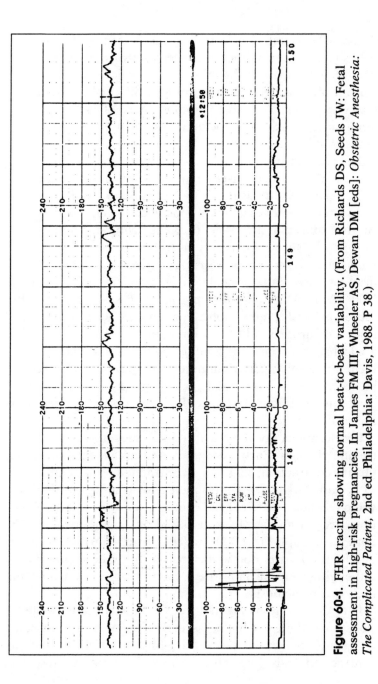

Figure 60-1. FHR tracing showing normal beat-to-beat variability. (From Richards DS, Seeds JW: Fetal assessment in high-risk pregnancies. In James FM III, Wheeler AS, Dewan DM [eds]: *Obstetric Anesthesia: The Complicated Patient*, 2nd ed. Philadelphia: Davis, 1988. P 38.)

decreased variability include drugs, such as atropine and narcotics given to the mother, fetal sleep states, and cardiac and CNS abnormalities in the fetus.

Fetal sinus tachycardia and bradycardia can be seen in several conditions. The most common cause of tachycardia is amnionitis, which can develop following premature rupture of the membranes; it usually is associated with maternal fever. Drugs such as cocaine can cross the placenta and stimulate the fetal CNS. Other causes include fetal hypoxia and anemia.

Sinus bradycardia is the initial response to acute asphyxia; the degree of bradycardia will depend on the level of hypoxia. Bradycardias that are severe (< 60 beats/minute) and persist in spite of vigorous interventions (repositioning mother, supplemental oxygen) are obstetric emergencies and indicate the need for immediate surgical delivery. Moderate bradycardias (100–120 beats/minute) with normal FHR variability usually represent head compression and are not associated with fetal acidosis. Paracervical blocks for vaginal delivery are associated with bradycardia beginning about 7 minutes after placement and resolving by 15 minutes. This bradycardia is felt to be secondary to direct fetal toxicity by the local anesthetic drug due to rapid fetal uptake. Routine supportive measures are recommended.

Decelerations are the fourth major category of fetal heart tracing changes. Early decelerations start with the onset of uterine contraction, peak as the contraction peaks, and return to baseline when the contraction ends (Fig. 60-2); they develop secondary to fetal head compression. Variable decelerations are variable in their onset and offset, although usually both are abrupt (Fig. 60-3). Under most circumstances, these decelerations are not associated with fetal compromise, although severe variable decelerations may indicate fetal hypoxia and acidosis.

Late decelerations are the most ominous. Late decelerations have the same shape as early decelerations but start after the contraction starts and return to baseline after the contraction ends (Fig. 60-4). These decelerations indicate

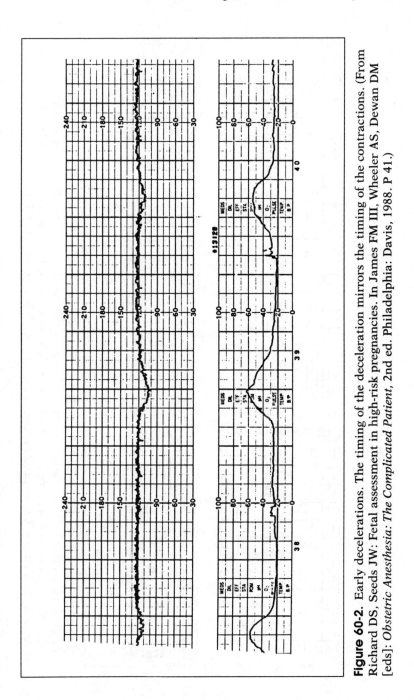

Figure 60-2. Early decelerations. The timing of the deceleration mirrors the timing of the contractions. (From Richard DS, Seeds JW: Fetal assessment in high-risk pregnancies. In James FM III, Wheeler AS, Dewan DM [eds]: *Obstetric Anesthesia: The Complicated Patient*, 2nd ed. Philadelphia: Davis, 1988. P 41.)

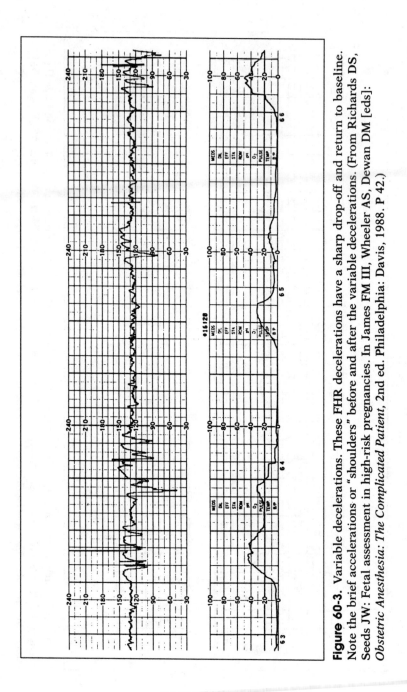

Figure 60-3. Variable decelerations. These FHR decelerations have a sharp drop-off and return to baseline. Note the brief accelerations or "shoulders" before and after the variable decelerations. (From Richards DS, Seeds JW: Fetal assessment in high-risk pregnancies. In James FM III, Wheeler AS, Dewan DM [eds]: *Obstetric Anesthesia: The Complicated Patient,* 2nd ed. Philadelphia: Davis, 1988. P 42.)

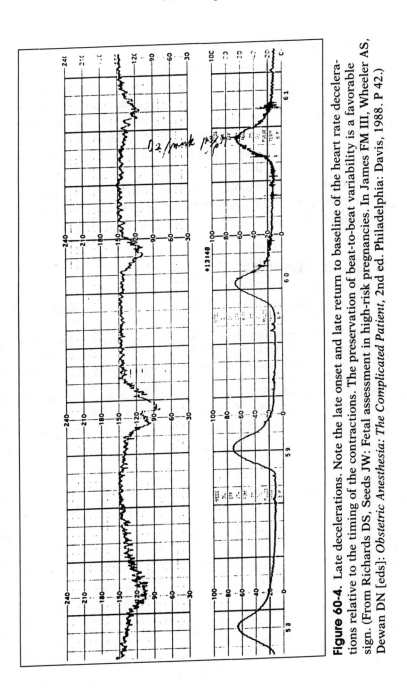

Figure 60-4. Late decelerations. Note the late onset and late return to baseline of the heart rate decelerations relative to the timing of the contractions. The preservation of beat-to-beat variability is a favorable sign. (From Richards DS, Seeds JW: Fetal assessment in high-risk pregnancies. In James FM III, Wheeler AS, Dewan DN [eds]: *Obstetric Anesthesia: The Complicated Patient*, 2nd ed. Philadelphia: Davis, 1988. P 42.)

uteroplacental insufficiency and direct fetal myocardial hypoxic depression. Correctable causes include (1) uterine hyperstimulation (secondary to augmentation of labor by oxytocin) and (2) maternal hypotension (secondary to aorto-caval compression or following subarachnoid or epidural blockade) (see Chapter 62). Treatment includes ensuring uterine displacement, administering intravenous fluids and oxygen, and reducing the oxytocin infusion rate. If vascular abnormalities are present, such as in patients with diabetes mellitus or preeclampsia, it may indicate the need for early delivery of the fetus.

SELECTED READING

Finster M, Petrie RH: Monitoring the fetus. *Anesthesiology* 45 : 198, 1976.

Palmar S: What anesthesiologists should know about fetal monitoring and fetal distress. *41st Annual Refresher Course Lectures and Clinical Update Program*. American Society of Anesthesiologists. Lecture 531, pp 1–6.

Ralston DH, Shnider SM: The fetal and neonatal effects of regional anesthesia in obstetrics. *Anesthesiology* 48 : 34, 1978.

61
Hypertension During Pregnancy

DEFINITION

In an uncomplicated pregnancy, the blood pressure remains at prepregnancy values, since increases in cardiac output are balanced by decreases in peripheral vascular resistance. If the blood pressure increases to greater than 140/90 mm Hg, the patient is considered to have hypertension. The American College of Obstetrics and Gynecology recognizes four categories of hypertension: preeclampsia, chronic hypertension, chronic hypertension with superimposed preeclampsia, and late or transient hypertension. For anesthetic purposes, causes of hypertension during pregnancy can be divided into three categories: (1) preexisting, (2) pregnancy induced, and (3) drug related.

ETIOLOGY
  I. Preexisting
     A. Essential hypertension
     B. Coarctation of the aorta
     C. Pheochromocytoma
     D. Autonomic hyperreflexia
     E. Renal disease
     F. Cushing's disease
     G. Hyperaldosteronism
 II. Pregnancy induced
     A. Pregnancy-induced hypertension (preeclampsia)
     B. Trophoblastic disease (molar pregnancy)
III. Drug related
     A. Illicit drugs (cocaine, amphetamines)

B. Ergot alkaloids
C. Epinephrine
D. Drug withdrawal (alcohol, antihypertensive medication)

DISCUSSION

A review of the patient's medical record will help rule out many causes of hypertension. Hypertension occurs in 6 percent of all pregnancies, with preexisting hypertension accounting for 25 percent of these cases (see Chapter 14). Essential hypertension or hypertension secondary to renal disease is usually diagnosed prior to pregnancy. A parturient with paraplegia and a spinal cord lesion higher than T6 may have autonomic hyperreflexia triggered by either a distended bladder or insufficient anesthesia for labor. Coarctation of the aorta can essentially be ruled out by measuring the blood pressure in both arms and by comparing the amplitude of the radial to femoral pulses. Other rare causes of preexisting hypertension include pheochromocytoma, hyperaldosteronism, and Cushing's disease.

Pregnancy-induced hypertension develops in 5 to 10 percent of all pregnancies and accounts for 40 percent of obstetric-related maternal deaths. It is called gestational hypertension when (1) the blood pressure is greater than 140/90 mm Hg in a previously normotensive patient or (2) either the systolic pressure is 30 mm Hg or the diastolic pressure is 15 mm Hg above prepregnant values. Preeclampsia is gestational hypertension with proteinuria or edema. In the majority of cases, pregnancy-induced hypertension develops after the twentieth gestational week; hypertension prior to the twentieth week suggests a molar pregnancy.

The third category of hypertension is drug related. With the high prevalence of drug use in society, the new onset of hypertension in a previously normotensive individual may indicate either recent cocaine or amphetamine ingestion or alcohol withdrawal. Abrupt withdrawal of antihypertensive medication, particularly beta-blocking agents or clonidine, may precipitate an acute hypertensive crisis. During labor, epinephrine added to local anesthetics for test dosing epidural catheters may lead to a transient elevation in blood pressure, particularly in a previously hypertensive patient. Ergot alkaloids given postpartum to augment uterine contraction can produce severe hypertension, especially when combined with vasopressor medication. The effect is so profound that ergot compounds should not be used in hypertensive patients in conjunction with vasopressors.

SELECTED READING

Lechner RB, Chadwick HS: Anesthetic care of the patient with preeclampsia. *Anesthesiol Clin North Am* 8 : 95, 1990.
Lindheimer MD, Katz AI: Hypertension in pregnancy. *N Engl J Med* 313 : 675, 1985.

62
Maternal Hypotension

DEFINITION

Hypotension is defined as a decrease in the blood pressure below baseline levels. In the healthy pregnant patient, the blood pressure remains at values similar to prepregnancy levels; significant decreases in pressure can cause problems for both the mother and the fetus. Hypotension is caused by a variety of disorders, including decreased venous return, hypovolemia, and miscellaneous factors (see Chapter 13).

ETIOLOGY

   I. Decreased venous return
      A. Aortocaval compression (supine hypotension syndrome)
      B. Regional anesthesia (epidural, subarachnoid blockade)
  II. Hypovolemia
      A. Hyperemesis
      B. Hemorrhage (abruptio placentae, placenta previa)
      C. Pregnancy-induced hypertension
 III. Miscellaneous factors
      A. Cardiac disease (cardiomyopathy, mitral stenosis)
      B. Drugs (antihypertensive medication, diuretics)

DISCUSSION

Before diagnostic studies begin, hypotension in the pregnant patient should be treated aggressively, particularly if associated with changes in the fetal heart tracing (see Chap. 60); if left untreated, permanent damage to the fetus may occur. Initial interventions should include rapid administration of intravenous fluid and ensuring left lateral uterine displacement. Early treatment of maternal hypotension may attenuate the decline in fetal pH.

The next step is to review the patient's history and medication record. The patient may give a history of protracted vomiting or use of diuretics to combat pedal edema. She may have known valvular heart disease, such as mitral stenosis, although rarely does it initially present in late pregnancy. Pregnancy-associated cardiomyopathy usually develops in the postpartum period.

When hypotension occurs suddenly, it may be due to (1) aortocaval compression, (2) sudden onset of sympathectomy secondary to regional anesthesia, or (3) maternal hemorrhage. Hypotension due to epidural or subarachnoid anesthesia may be exaggerated in patients with pregnancy-induced hypertension, since these patients are hypovolemic secondary to chronic vasoconstriction. Hypotension may be attenuated by adequate volume loading prior to instituting regional anesthesia. Maternal hemorrhage may be obvious, as with profound vaginal bleeding secondary to placenta previa, or occult, as when an abruption occurs; however, abruption is usually associated with severe abdominal pain.

SELECTED READING

Corke BC: Complications of obstetric anesthesia. In James FM III, Wheeler AS, Dewan DM (eds): *Obstetric Anesthesia: The Complicated Patient*, 2nd ed. Philadelphia: Davis, 1988. Pp 113–130.

Wright RG, Shnider SM: Hypotension and regional anesthesia. In Shnider SM, Levinson G (eds): *Anesthesia for Obstetrics*, 2nd ed. Baltimore: Williams & Wilkins, 1987. Pp 293–299.

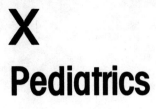

X
Pediatrics

63
Postoperative Apnea in Infants

DEFINITION

Apnea is defined as (1) unexplained cessation of breathing for longer than 20 seconds or (2) a shorter respiratory pause when associated with bradycardia, cyanosis, or pallor. Apnea commonly occurs after general anesthesia in premature infants and former "preemies," while it rarely occurs in term infants. The newborns at greatest risk are those less than 44 weeks postconceptual age who have a history of either prematurity or apnea and bradycardia. Causes of apnea can be divided into two categories: (1) metabolic disturbances and (2) central nervous system (CNS) disorders.

ETIOLOGY
  I. Metabolic
     A. Hypothermia
     B. Hypoglycemia
     C. Hypocalcemia
     D. Hypoxemia
     E. Respiratory acidosis
     F. Sepsis
 II. Central nervous system
     A. Residual drug effects (anesthetic agents)
     B. Congenital anomalies
     C. Intraventricular hemorrhage
     D. Idiopathic apnea of infancy

DISCUSSION

Apnea after general anesthesia or regional anesthesia with sedation is caused by metabolic derangements or immaturity of the CNS, combined with the depressant effects of residual anesthetic agents. Metabolic derangements include hypothermia, hypoglycemia, hypocalcemia, respiratory acidosis, and hypoxemia. In premature infants, indolent sepsis should be considered; diagnosing sepsis is difficult in this group and is often based on the findings of apnea, temperature instability, hypoglycemia, and an elevated white blood cell count. Therefore, when apnea occurs, laboratory studies that should be evaluated include complete blood count, serum electrolytes, arterial blood gases, and serum glucose.

CNS immaturity or congenital anomalies are the second major predisposing factor for postoperative apnea. It is probably due to the immaturity of the respiratory control center. Intraventricular hemorrhage, a common finding in premature infants, increases the risk of apnea; it can be diagnosed by computed tomography (CT) scan or cranial ultrasound.

Both metabolic and CNS disorders are exacerbated by the depressant effects of anesthetic compounds, since most drugs used affect respiration, either directly or indirectly. The effect of both hypoxemia and hypercarbia on the respiratory center is blunted by low concentrations of volatile anesthetic agents. In addition, most anesthetic drugs decrease muscle tone in the upper airway, which can lead to upper airway obstruction, labored breathing, fatigue, and ultimately apnea following surgery (Fig. 63–1). In premature infants, centrally acting drugs, such as narcotics or sedatives, should be avoided when possible; in fact, the benefit of regional over general anesthesia on postoperative apnea is virtually eliminated when sedation is given with regional anesthesia. The administration of intravenous caffeine has been shown to reduce episodes of postoperative apnea dramatically in premature infants.

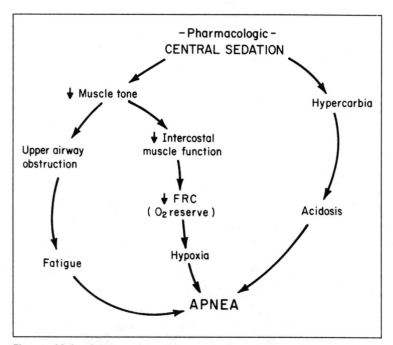

Figure 63-1. Pharmacologic interventions may result in several sequences of events. (From Coté CJ, Todres ID, Ryan JF: The preoperative evaluation of pediatric patients. In Ryan JF, Coté CJ, Todres ID, et al [eds]: *A Practice of Anesthesia for Infants and Children* Orlando: Grune & Stratton, 1986.)

SELECTED READING

Cox RG, Goresky GV: Life-threatening apnea following spinal anesthesia in former premature infants. *Anesthesiology* 73 : 345, 1990.

Welborn LG, Rice LS, Hannallah RS, et al: Postoperative apnea in former preterm infants: Prospective comparisons of spinal and general anesthesia. *Anesthesiology* 72 : 838, 1990.

64
Cyanotic Newborn

DEFINITION

Cyanosis, defined as a bluish discoloration of the skin, lips, or mucous membranes, may be central or peripheral. Central cyanosis, due to either arterial desaturation or abnormal hemoglobin, causes the tongue and mucous membranes to be blue. The peripheral form is secondary to an increased amount of reduced hemoglobin in venous blood with normal arterial oxygen saturation; it is also called acrocyanosis (*acro* meaning "extremity"), since it is confined to the hands and feet. While acrocyanosis is common in healthy newborns, central cyanosis indicates more serious pathology. Causes of central cyanosis fall into three categories: (1) cardiac disorders, (2) respiratory disorders, and (3) abnormal forms of hemoglobin.

ETIOLOGY
I. Central cyanosis
   A. Cardiac disorders
      1. Cyanotic congenital heart disease (transposition of great vessels, tetralogy of Fallot)
      2. Pulmonary arteriovenous fistula
   B. Respiratory disorders
      1. Respiratory distress syndrome
      2. Persistent fetal circulation
      3. Aspiration (meconium, tracheoesophageal fistula)
      4. Pneumothorax
      5. Central respiratory depression (narcotics, intracranial hemorrhage, intrauterine hypoxia)

      6. Neuromuscular dysfunction (drugs)
      7. Upper airway obstruction (macroglossia, congenital vascular ring)
      8. Diaphragmatic hernia
   C. Abnormal forms of hemoglobin
      1. Methemoglobinemia (familial, acquired)
      2. Low oxygen affinity hemoglobin variants (hemoglobin Kansas)
II. Peripheral
   A. Poor peripheral circulation (congestive heart failure, shock)
   B. Cold stress
   C. Polycythemia

DISCUSSION

Peripheral cyanosis occurs in nearly all newborns and usually resolves shortly after administering oxygen and warming the infant. If cyanosis persists after these measures, further diagnostic steps should be taken. Patients with polycythemia (hematocrit greater than 65%) may have peripheral cyanosis. Polycythemia can occur in infants (1) small for gestational age, (2) with chromosomal abnormalities (trisomy 21 or Down's syndrome), and (3) following twin-twin transfusions. Rarely, neonates will have acrocyanosis secondary to shock or congestive heart failure.

Central cyanosis is primarily due to a large amount of reduced hemoglobin in arterial blood; in a newborn it can be clinically detected when either 5 g of reduced hemoglobin or an oxygen saturation of 75 to 88 percent is present. The initial workup should include arterial blood gases (ABGs), chest radiograph, and hematocrit. ABGs may be helpful in distinguishing pulmonary from cardiac disorders. In both cases, the arterial oxygen tension is low. However, in patients with cyanosis secondary to pulmonary disease, some improvement occurs when 100% oxygen is administered; oxygen therapy does not help newborns with right-to-left shunts, since blood bypasses the alveoli. In addition, the arterial carbon dioxide level is normal with right-to-left shunts of congenital heart lesions, while it is usually elevated in pulmonary disorders. A chest radiograph may reveal cardiomegaly or altered pulmonary vascular markings in infants with congenital heart disease or may show a ground-glass appearance in newborns with respiratory distress syndrome. The hematocrit may be elevated secondary to chronic tissue hypoxia.

Severe cyanosis and tachypnea without apparent respiratory distress (i.e., retractions, stridor) indicate congenital heart disease. Transposition of the great vessels, the most common cause of cyanotic congenital heart disease in infants, presents in the first 2 to 3 days of life. Tetralogy of Fallot produces cyanosis at birth in one-third of patients with this abnormality; however, in two-thirds it does not appear until the child begins to walk or run. Other causes of cyanotic congenital heart disease presenting at birth include tricuspid atresia, hypoplastic left heart syndrome, and pulmonary atresia. An echocardiogram or cardiac catheterization is indicated to establish a diagnosis.

Persistent fetal circulation leads to cyanosis, tachypnea, and acidemia in the first few days of life in a term or near-term infant. It results from persistent pulmonary hypertension with subsequent shunting of blood through the foramen ovale or ductus arteriosus. It can develop following meconium aspiration, hypoglycemia, or asphyxia or in infants small for gestational age. ABGs drawn simultaneously from the umbilical and right radial arteries may show an oxygen tension difference greater than 10 mm Hg. An ultrasound of the heart reveals normal cardiac anatomy.

A variety of disorders affecting the lungs or respiratory center may lead to cyanosis. In premature infants, the lack of surfactant in the immature alveoli leads to atelectasis and subsequently respiratory distress syndrome; it rarely occurs in infants greater than 36 weeks gestational age, since a sufficient amount of surfactant is produced by this time. Other disorders in premature or stressed infants include meconium aspiration and failure of the central respiratory center; the latter may be secondary to prematurity itself, intracranial hemorrhage, or intrauterine hypoxia. Drugs administered to the mother may cross the placenta and affect the infant; these medications include narcotics, which directly depress the neonatal respiratory center, and diazepam, which produces hypotonia.

Certain congenital anomalies increase the likelihood of cyanosis in the neonate. Aspiration is a frequent finding in infants with tracheoesophageal fistulas. Upper airway obstruction may be due to macroglossia or vascular rings. A diaphragmatic hernia leads to hypoxemia and cyanosis for two reasons: (1) the left lung is hypoplastic secondary to direct compression by the abdominal contents and (2) the right lung is hypoplastic, since it was compressed by the mediastinum which had shifted into the right hemithorax. It is often diagnosed in utero with prenatal ultrasound; physical findings at birth include a scaphoid abdomen and bowel sounds in the left hemithorax.

The third cause of cyanosis is abnormal forms of hemoglobin. Methemoglobinemia may be either familial or acquired; the blood is chocolate brown and does not become red when mixed with air. For patients to be cyanotic, methemoglobin must compose at least 15 percent (1.5–2.0 g/dl) of the total hemoglobin. Diagnosis is made by CO-oximetry of an arterial blood sample. Acquired forms may be due to benzocaine ointment or aniline dyes found in some diapers. Lastly, low-oxygen affinity hemoglobin variants, such as hemoglobin Kansas, are associated with cyanosis and chronic tissue hypoxia.

SELECTED READING

Bellet PS: *The Diagnostic Approach to Common Symptoms and Signs in Infants, Children, and Adolescents.* Philadelphia: Lea & Febiger, 1989. Pp 73–78.

Kitterman JA: Cyanosis in the newborn infant. *Pediatr Rev* 4 : 13, 1982.

Pearse LA, Schaffer MS. *Handbook of Pediatrics*, 16th ed. Norwalk, CT: Appleton & Lange, 1991. Pp 604–609.

XI
Postanesthesia Care Unit

65
Delirium/Agitation

DEFINITION

Delirium is defined as a mental disturbance of short duration, characterized by cerebral excitement, incoherence, delusions, hallucinations, and physical hyperactivity, while agitation is a milder state of restlessness and mental distress. When these states occur at the end of general anesthesia, they are referred to as emergence delirium. Although commonly due to residual anesthetic effects, other conditions that can cause delirium or agitation should be excluded. These conditions can be divided into two categories: (1) respiratory and (2) other causes.

ETIOLOGY

I. Respiratory
   A. Hypoxemia
   B. Hypercarbia
   C. Upper airway obstruction
   D. Residual muscle relaxants
II. Other
   A. Urinary distention
   B. Gastric distention
   C. Pain
   D. Anxiety/psychological factors
   E. Drugs (sedatives, anticholinergics, ketamine, phenothiazines, "street" drugs)
   F. Surgical procedure (tonsillectomy, thyroid and middle ear surgery)

    G. Increased intracranial pressure
    H. Hyponatremia
    I. Hyperthyroidism
    J. Drug withdrawal (alcohol, narcotic, barbiturate)
    K. Organic brain syndrome
    L. Hyperosmolar states (uncontrolled diabetes mellitus or diabetes insipidus)

DISCUSSION

While the cause of agitation is being investigated, care must be taken to prevent patients from injuring themselves or others. Initially, sedatives should be avoided since dysphoric reactions are common, particularly in the elderly; therefore, manual restraints may be needed. At the same time, the adequacy of the patient's gas exchange should be evaluated. Hypoxemia, hypercapnia, airway obstruction, and partial paralysis can produce marked agitation. Arterial blood gases and/or pulse oximetry should be monitored while supplemental oxygen is administered. A peripheral nerve stimulator may reveal weakness due to residual muscle relaxants; additional reversal agents or reintubation with assisted ventilation may be required.

Urinary and gastric distention are frequent causes of postoperative agitation. Urinary retention occurs more commonly in elderly males and in those patients who received subarachnoid or epidural anesthesia. Relief of the distention will usually lead to prompt resolution of the agitated state.

Other common causes of agitation include pain and anxiety. If a patient is unable to voice complaints, the only indications of pain may be agitation, tachycardia, and hypertension; this condition usually responds to intravenous narcotics. Anxiety may be another contributor, particularly in younger individuals who were apprehensive about the operative findings. Reassurance is often all that is needed; in addition, small doses of sedatives, such as midazolam, may be beneficial.

Many drugs can cause delirium, which may be initially present in the recovery room. They include preoperative medications such as scopolamine, droperidol, phenothiazines, and barbiturates. Geriatric patients, particularly those individuals with organic brain syndrome, are more sensitive to these drugs and have a greater risk of this side effect. Patients who have undergone emergency surgery, particularly for trauma, may have taken unknown types or amounts of "street" drugs preoperatively. Ketamine and atropine given intraoperatively may also produce delirium; physostigmine may reverse agitation due to anticholinergics.

The surgical procedure itself may lead to agitation. Tonsillectomies and thyroid surgery have been reported to have a high incidence of postoperative agitation. Middle ear surgery is associated with restlessness, probably due to disturbances of the labyrinthine system. Increased intracranial pressure may develop in trauma or neurosurgical patients. Lastly, hyponatremia following transurethral resection of the prostate may present as altered mental status.

Preoperative conditions that may predispose to agitation include hyperthyroidism, other endocrine disturbances, and drug withdrawal. Uncontrolled diabetes mellitus or diabetes insipidus may lead to a hyperosmolar state and subsequent confusion. Acute withdrawal in patients addicted to drugs such as alcohol or narcotics may first present in the recovery room following a protracted period of abstinence.

SELECTED READING

Rosenberg H: Postoperative emotional responses. In: *Complications in Anesthesiology*. Philadelphia: Lippincott, 1983. Pp 355–367.

66
Postoperative Hypertension

DEFINITION

Postoperative hypertension is defined as an elevation in the arterial blood pressure in the hours immediately following surgery. The exact value varies with age, although a level of 140/90 mm Hg or greater in an adult or a 20 to 30 percent elevation from the baseline blood pressure in a previously normotensive individual is usually considered hypertensive. Causes of postoperative hypertension can be divided into four categories: (1) preexisting, (2) anesthesia related, (3) procedure related, and (4) physiologic disturbances.

ETIOLOGY
   I. Preexisting—see Chap. 14
  II. Anesthesia related
   A. Drug effects
      1. Administration (vasopressors, naloxone, anti-cholinergics, monoamine [MAO] oxidase inhibitors + meperidine or ephedrine)
      2. Withdrawal (antihypertensive medication, narcotics, alcohol)
   B. Anxiety
   C. Endotracheal intubation
   D. Shivering
   E. Emergence delirium
   F. Factitious
 III. Procedure related
   A. Pain
   B. Post–coarctation of the aorta repair

C. Post–carotid endarterectomy
D. Post–aortocoronary bypass grafting
E. Post–aortic valve replacement
F. Post–abdominal aortic aneurysm surgery
G. Postpartum hypertension (preeclampsia)
H. Increased intracranial pressure (ICP)
IV. Physiologic disturbances
A. Hypoxia
B. Hypercarbia
C. Hypoglycemia
D. Hypervolemia (blood, crystalloid)
E. Autonomic hyperreflexia
F. Distended bladder
G. Hypothermia

DISCUSSION

In the postoperative period, hypertension should be aggressively controlled to prevent complications such as bleeding from arterial or venous suture lines, excessive third-space fluid losses, myocardial ischemia or infarction, or intracranial hemorrhage or hypertension. The consequences depend not only on the degree of elevation but also on the underlying problem producing hypertension. In most cases, the elevated blood pressure should be treated while the underlying cause is being investigated.

Once factitious causes of hypertension have been excluded (blood pressure cuff too small for the extremity, arterial line overshoot), respiratory depression should be excluded, since both hypoxia and hypercarbia stimulate the sympathetic nervous system, resulting in hypertension. Supplemental oxygen should be administered as pulse oximetry or arterial blood gases are monitored. Patients who had intracranial surgery or sustained major head trauma are at increased risk for elevated ICP. If hypertension develops in these patients, an elevated ICP should be suspected, since hypertension is a physiologic response to maintain cerebral perfusion pressure. Neuro-surgical consultation should be requested as interventions to decrease ICP are instituted.

The most common causes of postoperative hypertension are poorly controlled preoperative hypertension and pain. Essential hypertension accounts for 95 percent of all cases; many patients have inadequate treatment (if any at all) prior to surgery. In addition, the abrupt withdrawal of anti-hypertensive medication such as clonidine or propranolol during the perioperative period may present as rebound hypertension in the postanesthesia care unit. Pain triggers a sympathoadrenal response with catecholamine release and increased blood pressure. Other causes of discomfort, such as a distended bladder, will produce a similar reaction.

Other physiologic disturbances that can produce hyper-tension include hypoglycemia, hypervolemia, hypothermia, and autonomic hyperreflexia. Hypoglycemia triggers cate-cholamine release, which leads to tachycardia, hypertension, and tremulousness (see Chap. 46). Hypervolemia and hypo-thermia are usually more contributory than causative. In patients with end-stage renal disease, blood pressure is often directly related to volume status, and hypertension may be corrected with adequate dialysis. Hypertension secondary to hypothermia is aggravated by shivering. Autonomic hyper-reflexia can develop in patients with spinal cord lesions at T6 or higher; the lesion may be secondary to various insults, including trauma and multiple sclerosis. A potent stimulus, such as distention of a hollow viscus (bladder, bowel), leads to sympathetic discharge that cannot be influenced by central inhibitory neurons; the result is profound hypertension.

Certain surgical procedures are associated with a high inci-dence of postoperative hypertension. Abnormal baroreceptor function following a carotid endarterectomy may lead to hypertension in up to 20 percent of patients. Spontaneous correction of hypertension following aortic valve replacement or coarctation repair may take days to weeks, if it occurs at all. It often takes several days for postpartum hypertension to resolve following delivery of the fetus. Aortocoronary bypass surgery and replacement of an abdominal aortic aneurysm are routinely followed by hypertension.

Drugs play a role in postoperative hypertension in several ways. There may be medication errors; for example, a patient may be receiving an intravenous vasopressor, such as phenyl-ephrine, without the recovery room nurse's knowledge. Patients taking MAO inhibitors have an exaggerated response to indirect sympathomimetics, such as ephedrine and mepe-ridine; it may develop if the MAO inhibitors have not been withdrawn at least 2 to 3 weeks before elective surgery. Cocaine administered intraoperatively may affect blood pressure postoperatively. Withdrawal of alcohol or narcotics in patients habituated to these compounds may precipitate hypertension; in addition, narcotic withdrawal may acutely develop if naloxone is given at the end of an anesthetic.

Several other conditions in the postanesthesia care unit can contribute to hypertension. Endotracheal intubation is a potent stimulus, particularly if the tip of the tube is irritating the carina. Patients may experience anxiety if the preoperative surgical diagnosis was uncertain. Emergence delirium may be due to pain, anxiety, or intraoperative treatment with anticholinergic drugs that cross the blood-brain barrier (atropine, scopolamine).

SELECTED READING

Davis R: Acute postoperative hypertension. *39th Annual Refresher Course Lectures and Clinical Update Program.* American Society of Anesthesiologists. Lecture 245, pp 1–6.

Faeley TW: Assessment and management of patients in the post-anesthesia care unit (PACU). *ASA Refresher Courses Anesthesiol* 18 : 149, 1990.

67
Hypoventilation

DEFINITION

Hypoventilation occurs when the rate of air movement into and out of the lungs is less than that necessary to maintain the blood carbon dioxide tension at the normal value. It leads to decreased carbon dioxide excretion and an increase in arterial carbon dioxide ($PaCO_2$). Rarely, the increased $PaCO_2$ is due to carbon dioxide overproduction, as can occur in malignant hyperthermia or postoperative shivering. Overall, the underlying causes of hypoventilation are (1) drug effects, (2) preexisting diseases, and (3) physical factors.

ETIOLOGY

I. Drug effects
   A. Narcotics (intravenous, neuroaxial)
   B. Sedatives
   C. Residual muscle relaxants
   D. Antibiotics (aminoglycosides)
   E. Inhalational anesthetics
   F. Magnesium sulfate ($MgSO_4$)
II. Preexisting diseases
   A. Chronic obstructive pulmonary disease (COPD)
   B. Neuromuscular disorders (myasthenia gravis, Guillain-Barré syndrome)
   C. Porphyria
   D. Neurologic insults (high cervical cord injury, cervical cordotomy)
   E. Brainstem lesions (trauma, hemorrhage)

III. Physical factors
   A. Hypothermia
   B. Prolonged hyperventilation
   C. Pain from high abdominal or thoracic incision
   D. Tight abdominal or thoracic strapping
   E. Pneumothorax
   F. Fractured ribs
   G. Increased work of breathing (upper airway obstruction, obesity)

DISCUSSION

The most common reason for alveolar hypoventilation in the postoperative period is residual anesthetic effects from narcotics, volatile agents, and sedatives. These drugs blunt the medullary respiratory center's responsiveness to carbon dioxide. Treatment includes assisted ventilation to excrete volatile anesthetics, incremental doses of naloxone to reverse narcotic effects, and intravenous flumazenil to counteract benzodiazepines. In trauma patients, drugs injected or ingested prior to injury may contribute to postoperative hypoventilation. Residual neuromuscular blockade may be secondary to inadequate doses of reversal agents, atypical pseudocholinesterase, phase II block, or potentiation of muscle relaxants by echothiophate or antibiotics. Additional reversal agents may help, but the effect is inconsistent when phase II block or antibiotics are the underlying problem. Other conditions that potentiate neuromuscular blockade include hypermagnesemia (from magnesium sulfate therapy for preeclampsia) and acute respiratory acidosis. Therefore, the acid-base balance and serum electrolytes should be evaluated and deviations corrected. If these measures are unsuccessful, intubation and mechanical ventilation may be necessary until the drugs are metabolized or excreted.

Preexisting diseases may directly contribute to alveolar hypoventilation. These diseases include (1) myasthenia gravis, particularly when muscle relaxants were administered, (2) porphyria, when sodium pentothal leads to a porphyric attack and subsequent neuromuscular weakness, and (3) Guillain-Barré syndrome. Patients with COPD who chronically retain carbon dioxide may hypoventilate when exposed to high levels of inspired oxygen, since their main stimulus for ventilation is arterial hypoxemia. When this stimulus is relieved, ventilation almost ceases (it should be noted that only a small percentage of patients with COPD have carbon dioxide retention). Rare neurologic causes of hypoventilation include cervical spinal cord injury and brainstem lesions. Failure of automatic ventilation following cervical cordotomy for chronic pain has been termed Ondine's curse, after the fairy whose human lover lost the ability to breathe automatically.

Physical factors may also lead to hypoventilation. High abdominal or thoracic incisions or rib fractures may cause shallow respirations secondary to pain. Tight abdominal or thoracic binders may physically impair normal tidal volumes. Hypothermia may potentiate anesthetic agents, including neuromuscular blocking drugs. Newborn and premature infants may become apneic when core temperature drops below 34.5°C, even in the absence of anesthetic drugs. Prolonged intraoperative hyperventilation may lead to loss of carbon dioxide from the body; as it slowly returns to normal postoperatively, the stimulus for breathing may be delayed. Other factors include pneumothorax and increased work of breathing secondary to obesity or upper airway obstruction. In addition, massive obesity may contribute if the patient has the obesity-hypoventilation, or pickwickian, syndrome. This rare condition can occur in patients who are morbidly obese (i.e., 100% over ideal body weight).

SELECTED READING

Feeley TW: Assessment and management of patients in the post-anesthesia care unit (PACU). *ASA Refresher Courses Anesthesiol* 18 : 149, 1990.
Pesola G, Kuetan V: Ventilatory and pulmonary problem management. *Anesthesiol Clin North Am* 8 : 284, 1990.

68
Postoperative Respiratory Failure

DEFINITION

Respiratory failure is defined as an impairment of gas exchange which leads to significant alterations in the arterial blood gases. Patients may have an arterial carbon dioxide tension ($PaCO_2$) greater than 50 mm Hg, an arterial oxygen tension (PaO_2) less than 50 mm Hg, or a combination of both. Since many cases of respiratory failure are not caused by pulmonary diseases, the responsible organ system needs to be identified. Causes can be divided into central nervous system, neuromuscular, thoracic, and pulmonary disorders.

ETIOLOGY

I. Central nervous system
  A. Head trauma
  B. Increased intracranial pressure (tumor, edema)
  C. Intracranial hemorrhage or infarction
  D. Infections (meningitis, encephalitis)
  E. Drugs (sedatives, anesthetic agents, narcotics)
  F. Seizures
  G. Hypothermia
II. Neuromuscular
  A. Cervical cord lesion
  B. Infections (Guillain-Barré syndrome, poliomyelitis, botulism)
  C. Myasthenia gravis
  D. Neurodegenerative diseases (muscular dystrophy, Werdnig-Hoffman paralysis, amyotrophic lateral sclerosis)

    E. Phrenic nerve injury
    F. Drugs (residual muscle relaxants, aminoglycosides)
    G. Electrolyte disturbances (hypophosphatemia, neonatal hypocalcemia)
III. Thoracic
    A. Kyphoscoliosis
    B. Flail chest
    C. Pneumothorax
    D. Large pleural effusions
    E. Severe abdominal distention
    F. Thoracic/upper abdominal incisions
    G. Obesity
    H. Ankylosing spondylitis
IV. Pulmonary
    A. Chronic obstructive pulmonary disease
    B. Airway obstruction (tumor, laryngospasm, vocal cord paralysis, foreign body, mucous plug)
    C. Asthma
    D. Pneumonia
    E. Pulmonary edema (cardiogenic, noncardiogenic, postobstructive)
    F. Massive atelectasis (endobronchial intubation)
    G. Pulmonary embolism (blood clot, fat, amniotic fluid)
    H. Pulmonary contusion
    I. "Shock" lung
    J. Acid aspiration
    K. Oxygen toxicity
    L. Smoke/chemical inhalation
    M. Cystic fibrosis

DISCUSSION

The preoperative history and physical examination will often identify patients who are at high risk for postoperative respiratory failure. Patients with significant central nervous system lesions (trauma, hemorrhage, tumor, infection) may have impaired control of ventilation due to the lesion itself, to increased intracranial pressure, or to generalized seizures. Trauma victims may have ingested drugs that depress ventilation; in addition, these patients may have a flail chest, pulmonary contusion, acid aspiration, or smoke inhalation. Neuromuscular disorders, such as myasthenia gravis, amyotrophic lateral sclerosis, and muscular dystrophy, may lead to respiratory failure, particularly when muscle relaxants have been given. Impairment of thoracic cage movement occurs in patients with severe kyphoscoliosis, obesity, or ankylosing spondylitis; these patients may be unable to generate adequate tidal volumes. Patients with severe preexisting lung disease are more prone to postoperative respiratory insufficiency; preoperative pulmonary function tests may identify patients at risk and allow for optimization of their pulmonary status (clearing secretions, treatment with bronchodilators or antibiotics) prior to surgery.

Following general anesthesia and surgery, a number of factors can interact to contribute to respiratory failure. Most anesthetic agents, including volatile gases, narcotics, and sedatives, can cause central respiratory depression. Residual effects of these compounds can affect normal individuals but are more pronounced in patients with underlying risk factors. Incomplete reversal of muscle relaxants is a common, and fully treatable, cause of respiratory insufficiency; the adequacy of reversal should be evaluated with a peripheral nerve stimulator or clinically by demonstrating sustained head lift for 5 seconds. Rarely, patients who were difficult to intubate may have sustained a cervical cord injury, which initially presents as failure to breathe postoperatively. Postobstructive pulmonary edema can develop after severe laryngospasm.

The site of surgery itself can play an important role in the patient's postoperative respiratory status. Thoracic or upper abdominal incisions often produce severe pain, resulting in hypoventilation; upper abdominal incisions can lead to decreases in tidal volume by up to 60 percent. Thyroid surgery can be associated with injury to the recurrent laryngeal nerves and subsequent vocal cord paralysis (see Chapter 3).

Patients may have phrenic nerve paralysis after open heart surgery due to thermal injury of the nerve produced by ice.

Other events that occur in the operating room can contribute to postoperative respiratory failure. Hypothermia, with core temperatures less than 34.5°C, not only impairs drug metabolism but may directly inhibit respiratory efforts, particularly in neonates. Patients who have received massive transfusions or large volumes of crystalloid may develop "shock" lung or pulmonary edema and require ventilatory support. An unrecognized endobronchial intubation may lead to atelectasis of an entire lung or lung segment. A variety of foreign bodies from endotracheal tubes and connectors have been retrieved from patients' airways after intubation. A pneumothorax may develop after attempts at subclavian vein cannulation, particularly when followed by positive-pressure ventilation.

Arterial blood gas analysis is mandatory, not only to diagnose respiratory failure but also to help determine the cause. Respiratory failure may be divided into hypercapnic or non-hypercapnic (hypoxemic) failure. Hypercapnic failure is associated with an elevated $PaCO_2$ and a decreased PaO_2. It usually results from hypoventilation secondary to extra-pulmonary disorders, ventilation-perfusion mismatching, or a combination of the two. Hypoxemic respiratory failure, with low PaO_2 and low-to-normal $PaCO_2$, results from pulmonary dysfunction or right-to-left shunting, but not from extrapulmonary disorders.

Other diagnostic studies will depend on the patient's underlying diseases. A chest radiograph can reveal pulmonary edema, pneumonia, atelectasis, or pneumothorax. Testing the patient's ability to generate a negative inspiratory force and forced vital capacity will help determine whether the problem is neuromuscular in origin. Severe hypophosphatemia can occur in patients receiving large glucose loads, as in total parenteral nutrition with inadequate phosphate supplementation, or when diabetic ketoacidosis is rapidly corrected; therefore, serum phosphate should be measured. Hypocalcemia may first present as apnea in neonates. Pulmonary artery catheterization may be necessary to distinguish cardiogenic from noncardiogenic pulmonary edema. Lastly, rigid or fiberoptic bronchoscopy is indicated if a foreign body or mucous plug is suspected.

SELECTED READING

Bready LL: Prolonged postoperative apnea. In Bready LL, Smith RB: *Decision Making in Anesthesiology*. Toronto: Decker, 1987. Pp 164–165.

Jordan C: Assessment of the effects of drugs on respiration. *Br J Anaesth* 54 : 763, 1982.

Schwieger I, Gamulin Z, Suter PM: Lung function during anesthesia and respiratory insufficiency in the postoperative period: Physiological and clinical implications. *Acta Anaesthesiol Scand* 33 : 527, 1989.

69
Prolonged Neuromuscular Blockade

DEFINITION

Both depolarizing and nondepolarizing muscle relaxants are administered intraoperatively for a wide variety of reasons. The effect of the depolarizing agent succinylcholine dissipates through rapid metabolism by the enzyme pseudocholinesterase. The actions of nondepolarizing relaxants are antagonized by anticholinesterase drugs given at the end of surgery to reverse the blockade. Several factors may interfere with the return of normal neuromuscular function, which will leave patients partially paralyzed in the recovery room. In general, these factors depend on whether a depolarizing or nondepolarizing drug was administered.

ETIOLOGY

I. Depolarizing muscle relaxant
   A. Atypical pseudocholinesterase
   B. Phase II block
   C. Deficiencies in normal pseudocholinesterase activity (echothiophate, anticholinesterase drugs)
II. Nondepolarizing muscle relaxants
   A. Intense neuromuscular blockade
   B. Inadequate dose of anticholinesterase drugs
   C. Residual volatile anesthetics
   D. Delayed excretion (renal insufficiency)
   E. Acute respiratory acidosis
   F. Hypothermia

G. Potentiation of blockade by other drugs (magnesium, furosemide, dantrolene, aminoglycosides)
H. Underlying neuromuscular disorder (myasthenia gravis, familial periodic paralysis)

DISCUSSION

As the cause for prolonged paralysis is being investigated, the patient's ventilation should be supported and arterial blood gases or pulse oximetry should be monitored. In addition, if the patient is awake, amnestic drugs, such as midazolam, may be given to help make the patient more comfortable.

Succinylcholine can produce prolonged blockade by three mechanisms. First, it can cause a phase II block; this problem should be considered when large doses of succinylcholine (greater than 6 mg/kg) have been given and when the response to tetanic stimulation with the peripheral nerve stimulator shows fade. Secondly, the patient may have atypical pseudocholinesterase which impairs succinylcholine's metabolism and leads to paralysis for several hours. This disorder is genetically transmitted and should be suspected if the patient reports a family history of prolonged paralysis or delayed emergence postoperatively. It can be diagnosed by ordering a dibucaine number; however, it usually takes several days to obtain results and therefore is not helpful in the acute situation. Lastly, anticholinesterase drugs (neostigmine, edrophonium) and echothiophate will inhibit normal pseudocholinesterase activity; giving even a small dose of succinylcholine after any of these agents can lead to neuromuscular blockade for 45 to 60 minutes.

Nondepolarizing drugs can cause prolonged blockade for several reasons. Either a relative overdose of the drug or an inadequate amount of reversal agent may have been given. The patient may (1) have an unsuspected underlying neuromuscular disorder (myasthenia gravis), (2) be receiving other drugs that potentiate the blockade (aminoglycoside antibiotics or magnesium sulfate), (3) have delayed drug excretion (renal insufficiency), or (4) be hypothermic. Acute respiratory acidosis can potentiate residual drug effect. This situation can trigger a vicious cycle, as respiratory acidosis leads to a potentiation of the neuromuscular blockade, which leads to impaired ventilation, which leads to further respiratory acidosis.

SELECTED READING

Ali HH: Monitoring of neuromuscular function and clinical interaction. *Clin Anaesthesiol* 3 : 447, 1985.

Sokoll MD, Gergis SD: Antibiotics and neuromuscular function. *Anesthesiology* 55 : 148, 1981.

70
Delayed Emergence/ Failure to Regain Consciousness

DEFINITION

Following general anesthesia, most patients regain consciousness within 15 minutes of arrival in the recovery room. If return to consciousness is prolonged (greater than 20–30 minutes), prompt evaluation and diagnosis are essential so that reversible conditions can be corrected. In general, delayed emergence is secondary to three basic causes: (1) drug effects, (2) metabolic disorders, and (3) neurologic disorders.

ETIOLOGY
  I. Drug effects
     A. Volatile anesthetics
     B. Narcotics (intravenous, neuroaxial)
     C. Sedatives
     D. Muscle relaxants
     E. Intoxication (alcohol, "street" drugs)
     F. Other drugs (clonidine, cimetidine, antihistamines)
 II. Metabolic disorders
     A. Hypoxia
     B. Hypercapnia
     C. Acidosis
     D. Hypoglycemia
     E. Hyperosmolar nonketotic coma
     F. Electrolyte disorders (hyponatremia, hypocalcemia, hypermagnesemia)
     G. Hypothermia

   H. Severe hyperthermia (malignant hyperthermia, heat stroke)
   I. Underlying organ dysfunction (renal, hepatic, endocrine)
III. Neurologic disorders
   A. Cerebral ischemia
   B. Cerebral hemorrhage
   C. Cerebral embolism
   D. Postanoxic encephalopathy
   E. Intracranial mass lesion
   F. Seizure disorder
   G. Increased intracranial pressure
   H. Preexisting obtundation

DISCUSSION

As evaluation of delayed emergence commences, one must be sure that the patient's airway is patent and that air exchange is adequate. If not, oxygenation and ventilation should be supported until adequate respiratory effort begins.

Preexisting organ dysfunction may contribute to delayed awakening for three reasons. First, the patient may have an altered level of consciousness preoperatively secondary to uremia, hepatic encephalopathy or central nervous system disease. Second, patients with hepatic, renal, or certain endocrine disorders (hypothyroidism, adrenal insufficiency) may have an increased sensitivity to depressant medications. Lastly, organ dysfunction may delay metabolism or excretion of anesthetic compounds. Increased sensitivity and delayed drug excretion commonly occur in the elderly.

The most frequent cause of delayed awakening is residual effects of volatile and intravenous anesthetic agents. Prolonged obtundation is more likely if the surgical procedure was long, if high inspired concentrations of volatile agents were used, if long-acting sedatives or narcotics were given as premedication, or if excessive doses of sedatives or narcotics were administered intraoperatively. Incremental low-dose naloxone can counteract depression secondary to narcotics. Intravenous physostigmine or flumazenil may reverse sedation secondary to inhalational agents and some sedatives (scopolamine and benzodiazepines). Profound neuromuscular paralysis should be excluded with a peripheral nerve stimulator. In addition, drugs taken preoperatively may contribute to delayed emergence from general anesthesia. These drugs include alcohol, "street" drugs (Quaaludes), antihistamines, cimetidine, and some centrally acting antihypertensive agents (clonidine, methyldopa).

Several metabolic disturbances can lead to delayed awakening or coma in the postoperative period. Laboratory studies that should be obtained include arterial blood gases, serum glucose, and serum electrolytes. Severe hypoxia may lead to either agitation or delayed awakening. Acute hypercapnia and associated respiratory acidosis induce cerebrospinal fluid and cerebral tissue acidosis, as carbon dioxide crosses the blood-brain barrier; the results are narcosis, depression, and coma. In addition, hypercapnia indicates alveolar hypoventilation and therefore delayed excretion of volatile anesthetic agents.

Hypoglycemia may occur in infants who did not receive glucose perioperatively, in diabetics who were given insulin or long-acting hypoglycemic agents preoperatively, or in patients with insulin-secreting tumors that are manipulated intraoperatively. If hypoglycemia is suspected, intravenous dextrose should be infused, even before laboratory results have returned. Severe hyperglycemia with hyperosmolar, nonketotic coma may develop in adults with uncontrolled diabetes mellitus. Serum electrolytes may reveal hyponatremia (after transurethral resection of the prostate), hypocalcemia (after thyroid or parathyroid surgery), or hypermagnesemia (after magnesium sulfate therapy for preeclampsia).

Both hypo- and hyperthermia can cause delayed emergence. Hypothermia reduces the metabolism of depressant medication, increases the tissue solubility of volatile anesthetics, and directly depresses the brain. Severe hyperthermia can result in loss of consciousness, as seen in heat stroke victims.

As laboratory studies are being obtained, a thorough neurologic evaluation should be performed. Focal neurologic findings may indicate cerebral hemorrhage (following head trauma or hypertensive crisis), ischemia or infarction (following intraoperative hypotension), or embolism (following sitting craniotomies or in patients with atrial fibrillation or a hypercoagulable state). Unrecognized brain tumors or uncontrolled seizure activity may also lead to delayed awakening. If the patient is recovering from intracranial surgery, other possibilities include cerebral edema, increased intracranial pressure, and pneumocephalus. Postanoxic encephalopathy can follow a cardiac arrest.

SELECTED READING

Breedy LL: Delayed emergence. In Bready LL, Smith RB: *Decision Making in Anesthesiology*. Toronto: Decker, 1987. Pp 166–167.

Denlinger JK: Prolonged emergence and failure to regain consciousness. In *Complications in Anesthesiology*. Philadelphia: Lippincott, 1983. Pp 368–378.

XII
Regional Anesthesia

71
Failed Regional Technique
Hillel I. Kashtan

DEFINITION

Inadequate anesthesia caused by a failed regional technique is distressing to patients, surgeons, and anesthesiologists. The ineffective block also discourages future acceptance by the patient, and in some cases the surgeon, of an excellent alternative to general anesthesia. The definition of a failed regional technique varies between studies (e.g., requirements for intravenous or inhalation agent supplementation); therefore, the percentage of successful blocks is difficult to measure. The differential diagnosis of regional nerve block failure is divided into problems with the patient, anesthetic technique, and anesthetic drugs administered.

ETIOLOGY
I. Patient
  A. Uncooperative (intoxicated, mentally retarded, anxious)
  B. Anatomy
    1. Distorted (previous surgery, trauma)
    2. Normal variant preventing needle or catheter placement
  C. Misinterpretation of sensation (pain versus touch)
II. Anesthetic technique
  A. Incorrect nerve block for surgery
  B. Incorrect needle placement (needle moves during or prior to injection)

    C. Paresthesia
      1. Patient's inability to communicate effectively
      2. Misinterpretation of paresthesia
    D. Nerve stimulator
      1. Electrode-skin contact
      2. Cathode versus anode
      3. Insulated versus uninsulated needle
III. Anesthetic drug
    A. Incorrect choice of agent
    B. Inadequate concentration
    C. pH (sodium metabisulfite, tissue [inflammation, infection])
    D. Inadequate volume

DISCUSSION

It is important to establish proper patient selection for a regional technique during the preoperative interview. An apprehensive or uncooperative individual is unlikely to tolerate the sensations associated with surgeries performed under neural blockade. Therefore, when a regional anesthetic is chosen, it is imperative to inform patients of the sensations they will experience during the placement of the block as well as in the peri- and postoperative periods. One major patient concern is the fear of being awake and aware during the operative procedure. These individuals should be reassured that the degree of sedation will be titrated to provide a comfortable intraoperative course with minimal or no recall. It cannot be stressed enough that a relaxed, well-informed, motivated patient will markedly increase the success of a nerve block.

Previous surgeries or accidents may scar or distort local anatomy. Normal anatomic barriers may also further reduce success. For example, the myriad of sacral formations produces several structural variations that make needle or catheter placement within the caudal canal virtually impossible. The anterior approach to the sciatic nerve is another case in which the anatomic relationship (i.e., between neural bundle and femur) may hamper the placement of local anesthetic in close proximity to the nerve.

Understanding the spread of local anesthetic and the limitations of the nerve block performed will reduce the incidence of inappropriate choice of neural blockade. For example, there are four different approaches to brachial plexus anesthesia, each with advantages and disadvantages. The interscalene technique preferentially blocks the C3–C4 cervical plexus as well as the superior and middle brachial plexus trunks (C5–C7). With this approach, the ulnar nerve is frequently not anesthetized. The supraclavicular and subclavian perivascular blocks result in virtually identical spread over all the nerves of the brachial plexus. Finally, the axillary technique often misses the musculocutaneous nerve, which has emerged from the sheath proximal to the injection site. Therefore, the interscalene block is more appropriate for surgery on the upper arm or shoulder, whereas the axillary approach is better suited for hand operations. Anesthesia for procedures below the fourth thoracic dermatome can often be provided by a subarachnoid or epidural block. During upper abdominal surgery, vagal response may be elicited from visceral traction as well as direct gastric compression, potentially increasing the risk of regurgitation. In these cases, it would be prudent not to perform the operation in an awake patient but to combine either regional technique with a light general anesthetic.

The anesthesiologist must understand local anatomy to extrapolate a three-dimensional picture of the underlying landmarks and structures, which provides an estimation of the approximate depth and location of the nerve fibers. During needle placement, the different resistances of various structures to needle insertion also assist in determining the tissue plane through which the tip has passed. Therefore, greater experience, knowledge, and technical skill of the anesthesiologist often allow more accurate needle placement.

When paresthesia is used to locate nerve bundles, effective communication and understanding are necessary between the individual performing the block and the patient. Many conditions, by impairing cooperation or impeding patient reliability, reduce success. Drug or alcohol intoxication, heavy premedication, mental retardation, and language barrier are several examples. On the other hand, it may be the anesthesiologist who misinterprets the information delivered by the patient. Paresthesia that results from sciatic nerve stimulation should radiate to the foot. Occasionally, periosteal pain, induced by needle insertion on the bony rim of the sciatic notch, will cause sensation to be referred to the thigh or calf. Stimulation of the suprascapular nerve during interscalene brachial plexus blockade will produce paresthesia to the scapula or shoulder joint. The novice, in both situations, may incorrectly inject local anesthetic at this juncture.

Peripheral nerve stimulators may enhance the performance of blocks, although this technique has several pitfalls. First, the positive lead should make good skin contact. Second, approximately four times as much current is required to stimulate peripheral nerves when the needle serves as the anode. The cathode, or negative lead, should preferentially be used for nerve stimulation. Third, uninsulated needles require more current for nerve stimulation than insulated ones (1.2 mA versus 0.5 mA, respectively). Insulating the shaft negates this problem by localizing current output at the tip and allowing accurate placement.

The choice of an appropriate local anesthetic agent depends on the desired block characteristics. If prolonged duration is required, bupivacaine or etidocaine should be injected. Lidocaine or chloroprocaine will maintain surgical anesthesia for a shorter duration with a rapid return of normal function. The type of nerve fiber to be blocked (sensory, motor, or autonomic) should also influence drug selection. Etidocaine produces a greater motor blockade compared to the intense analgesia obtained with bupivacaine. Increasing local anesthetic concentration will augment the degree of motor block.

Conversely, very dilute solutions may only prevent impulse conduction along autonomic fibers, with subsequent sensory sparing. In addition, the physical spread of local anesthetic assumes greater importance if the target nerve is distant from the injection site. In this situation, a small volume of solution may have limited diffusion to distal axons. Therefore, a minimum agent concentration and volume are necessary to accomplish the requirements for each surgical procedure. The addition of epinephrine to local anesthetic solutions increases not only the degree of motor block but also its intensity and duration. However, commercially available premixed solutions of epinephrine and local anesthetic contain sodium metabisulfite, which may result in decreased efficacy. This antioxidant lowers pH in the preparation, causing increased drug ionization. Consequently, the charged molecules are unable to penetrate the nerve membrane to access their site of action. This same mechanism reduces effectiveness in areas of inflammation and infection. Tissue pH is lowered by the formation of lactic and other acids, causing a shift of the local anesthetic dissociation reaction toward the acid form.

Finally, pain and temperature impulses are transmitted along A-delta and C fibers. Larger myelinated A-beta fibers are related to touch and pressure sensation. Therefore, differential neural blockade may produce a situation where pain is abolished, but touch, pressure, and proprioception remain intact. Upon surgical incision, anxious patients may misconstrue these perceptions as pain. Reassurance or a small intravenous dose of a rapidly acting anesthetic agent prior to stimulation will achieve the desired objective.

SELECTED READING

Cousins MJ, Bridenbaugh PO: *Neural Blockade*, 2nd ed. Philadelphia: Lippincott, 1988. Pp 332–335, 393–405.

Levy JH, Islas JA, Ghia JN: A retrospective study of the incidence and causes of failed spinal anesthetics in a university hospital. *Anesth Analg* 64 : 705, 1985.

72
Postoperative Peripheral Neuropathy

Hillel I. Kashtan

DEFINITION

Peripheral neuropathy is one of the most common perioperative neurologic complications. In three separate series, which included over 100,000 patients, the incidence of nerve palsy was approximately 0.1 percent. Interestingly, in many cases, patients had their surgeries under general anesthesia. In view of the multitude of potential etiologies, it is important to delineate when the nerve damage occurred, that is, in the pre-, intra-, or postoperative period.

ETIOLOGY

I. Preoperative
   A. Idiopathic
   B. Traumatic (trauma, compression, stretching, intramuscular injection)
   C. Metabolic (diabetes mellitus, uremia, chronic alcoholism, amyloidosis, porphyria, multiple myeloma)
   D. Nutritional deficiencies (vitamin B_{12}, thiamine)
   E. Infection (local neural infection, tetanus, infectious mononucleosis)
   F. Drugs and toxins (isoniazid, vincristine, nitrofurantoin, heavy metals [lead, mercury], organic chemicals)
   G. Miscellaneous (hereditary [cervical rib syndrome, Charcot-Marie-Tooth disease], multiple sclerosis, collagen vascular disease, sarcoidosis, carcinomatous neuropathies)

II. Intraoperative
   A. Positioning
   B. Surgical (trauma, tourniquet, tight casts)
   C. Anesthetic (muscle relaxants, neural blockade)
III. Postoperative
   A. Exacerbation of preexisting neurologic disease
   B. Injury (tight cast or bandage)

DISCUSSION

Nerve damage or disease, whether diagnosed or not, may exist prior to surgery. The preoperative differential diagnosis included in this chapter lists the more common etiologies. During trauma, the physical forces that either directly produce injury or result from sudden displacement of fracture fragments have the potential for damaging neuronal tissue. Central or peripheral nerve function may be impaired by direct blunt trauma, laceration, or severe traction, although a higher incidence of nerve palsy occurs following specific traumatic injuries. For example, there may be associated axillary nerve damage during anterior shoulder dislocation. A displaced humeral shaft fracture may also injure the axillary nerve. The common peroneal nerve, as it winds around the fibular neck, is especially vulnerable when the proximal fibula has been fractured, and is also at risk for ischemia caused by a tight cast or bandage. This injury will present as a foot drop with sensory alterations on the anterolateral aspect of the foot.

Several systemic disorders may influence nerve function. Thiamine deficiency produces noninflammatory degeneration of the myelin sheath. Muscle weakness and diminished deep tendon reflexes occur, but some individuals will develop sensory changes. The most common neurologic picture observed with diabetes mellitus is that of a peripheral polyneuropathy. Symptoms, often bilateral, include numbness, paresthesia, and pain. Therefore, during the preoperative interview, an attempt must be made to elicit neurologic symptomatology. When individuals present with a disease entity that has known neurologic manifestations (e.g., multiple sclerosis), the history and physical examination, from a medicolegal point of view, attain added importance. A neurologic examination in the area to be anesthetized by a regional technique provides baseline data with which to compare any postoperative complication. Preoperative electromyography and nerve conduction studies, if appropriate, may be considered.

During the operative period, incorrect patient positioning may contribute to traction or compression neuropathies. There are reported cases of injury secondary to malpositioning of almost every peripheral nerve. The loss of sensation during a regional or general anesthetic reduces the patient's ability to respond to such insults, which are not normally tolerated. Muscle relaxants, by reducing muscle tone, may increase the potential for injury by allowing extremes in extension and flexion. Tourniquet-induced neurologic injury, either by improper positioning or prolonged or extremely elevated pressures, occurs in approximately 1 in 8000 cases. Although a rare complication, it must be considered. The exact mechanism producing impairment is unknown, but it is most likely due to direct mechanical compression or nerve ischemia.

During the performance of a regional anesthetic technique, many anesthesiologists seek a paresthesia to locate nerves and nerve plexuses. Obtaining a paresthesia may increase the risk of neurologic sequelae during axillary brachial plexus blockade, particularly when a standard sharp (14-degree bevel angle) needle is used. Blunt needles (45-degree angle) produce significantly less fascicular damage than sharp needles. The short bevel appears to push the nerve away, whereas sharp needles may cut fibers. Although not clinically proven, the addition of epinephrine may increase the risk of neurologic sequelae once nerve injury has occurred, perhaps through reduction in neural blood flow. Therefore, neural lesions may be minimized by the use of blunt needles, avoiding intraneural injections, exercising proper technique, and possibly withholding epinephrine from the local anesthetic solution.

When a neurologic deficit presents in the postoperative period, the blame is often placed on the anesthetic. The patient's history should be reviewed to elicit diagnostic clues and potential contributing factors that may affect nerve function, specifically drug or toxin exposure, systemic illness, and preexisting neurologic disease. A thorough physical examination should then be performed with an emphasis on the affected region. Sensory, motor, and autonomic deficits are mapped out and recorded. The neurologic evaluation is important for several reasons. First, it allows documentation of the degree of alteration in comparison to the preoperative baseline status. Second, the location of the lesion (i.e., segmental versus peripheral) can often be ascertained by the abnormalities detected. Third, the information obtained aids in distinguishing mononeuropathic from multiple mono- or polyneuropathic lesions. The presence of multiple mono- or polyneuropathic features suggests a systemic pathologic process.

Biochemical tests are helpful in ruling out toxic or metabolic disorders. Other useful diagnostic tools include needle electromyography (EMG) and nerve conduction velocity (NCV) studies. EMG testing involves the placement of needle electrodes directly into muscle. Electrical potentials are then measured at rest and during muscle contraction. Denervation, due to the loss of motor units, causes discrete or limited groups of muscle fibers to cease functioning. EMG patterns characteristic of denervation are decreased motor unit potential, spontaneous electrical discharges, and positive denervation potentials. These features can be distinguished from myopathic lesions in which the total number of motor units are unchanged but individual muscle fibers within the units are destroyed. By determining the pattern of muscle involvement, EMG testing can assist in localizing the lesion site. In addition, the involvement of paraspinous or proximally innervated muscles indicates that nerve damage has occurred central to the plexus or peripheral nerve. Even more importantly, degeneration potentials do not appear until approximately 3 weeks after injury. Consequently, EMG, when performed in the immediate postoperative period, may help in differentiating a perioperative-induced neuropathy from one that may have been present prior to surgery. Nerve conduction studies offer further information regarding the site of nerve injury. Sensory and motor fibers are percutaneously stimulated at two separate locations along the nerve course, and conduction action potentials are recorded. NCV is then calculated based on the relationship between distance and conduction times. It is important to note that NCV data are based on surviving nerve fibers. Therefore, velocity is usually not reduced unless only a few or no fibers remain intact.

SELECTED READING

Kane RE: Neurologic deficits following epidural or spinal anesthesia. *Anesth Analg* 60 : 151, 1981.

Wedel D: Complications of regional anesthesia. *42nd Annual Refresher Course Lectures and Clinical Update Program.* American Society of Anesthesiologists. Lecture 136, pp 1–7.

XIII
Miscellaneous

73
Alterations in Anesthetic Requirements

Timothy N. Harwood

DEFINITION

Response to a drug varies either in pharmacokinetics (change in what happens to the drug in the body) or pharmacodynamics (changes in the effect a drug has on the body).

ETIOLOGY

I. Pharmacokinetic changes
  A. Increased drug metabolism
    1. Enzyme induction
      a. Concomitant medication therapy
      b. Nonmedical chemical abuse
    2. Genetic variation—rapid acetylators
    3. Increased hepatic blood flow (HBF)
      a. Improvement in cardiac output with therapy
      b. Phenobarbital-induced
  B. Decreased drug metabolism
    1. Decreased hepatic enzyme activity—concomitant medication therapy
    2. Genetic variation
      a. Slow acetylators
      b. Atypical pseudocholinesterase
    3. Decreased hepatocirculatory function
      a. Decreased HBF
      b. Hepatic insufficiency or failure

       4. Decreased renal elimination
         a. Decreased renal blood flow
         b. Renal insufficiency or failure
II. Changes in pharmacodynamics
    A. Increased anesthetic requirement
       1. Pathophysiologic states (hyperthermia, hypernatremia)
       2. Drug-associated changes (chronic alcohol ingestion)
    B. Decreased anesthetic requirement
       1. Pathophysiologic state (severe hypoxia, hypercapnia, hypothermia)
       2. Drug-associated changes (acute alcohol ingestion, alpha-methyldopa)

DISCUSSION

Numerous and complex factors determine what response the anesthesiologist can expect when administering drugs to a patient. While serum levels affect the response to a drug, the drug level itself results from a combination of its physicochemical properties relative to the physiologic state of the patient. These properties include lipid solubility, ionization, protein binding, and molecular size. Pathophysiologic changes that affect distribution include altered pH, changes in plasma protein concentrations, and disruptions in blood-organ barriers. Examples of these changes include (1) severe metabolic acidosis altering drug binding by albumin and severe liver disease with subsequent hypoproteinemia, (2) decreased drug binding, and (3) septicemia resulting in increased capillary permeability to drugs.

The liver is the primary site of drug metabolism, while the kidney's main contribution is the clearance of hydrophilic drugs or metabolites from the body. Hepatic metabolism of drugs involves four basic processes: oxidation, reduction, conjugation, and hydrolysis. The two most common processes employed in the metabolism of drugs are oxidation and conjugation by hepatic microsomal enzymes, the most important of which is the cytochrome P-450 system. Hydrolysis and glucuronide-conjugating enzymes reside in the liver as well as in the plasma and the gastrointestinal tract. Increased drug metabolism occurs primarily by induction of metabolizing enzymes. Only reduction and oxidation (redox) enzymes are inducible; therefore, enzyme induction does not affect drugs metabolized primarily by hydrolysis. More than 300 compounds are known to cause enzyme induction (Table 73-1).

If either the blood flow to or the function of metabolizing organs decreases, impairment of the drug metabolism may occur. Common examples of this phenomenon include the reduction in hepatic and renal blood flow observed during the administration of volatile anesthetics or the diminished HBF caused by cimetidine or propanolol. Hepatic and renal blood flows directly relate to perfusion pressure (mean arterial-venous pressures). In the liver, the only autoregulated flow is in the arterial system, which carries just 25 percent of the total HBF; therefore, HBF is largely pressure dependent. Table 73-2 lists some of the factors that affect HBF. Effects on the kidney are similar to those on the liver, although the kidney autoregulates its blood flow to a greater extent, and drugs do not directly affect its flow. For the most part, critical impairment in drug metabolic activity occurs only when severe hepatocellular dysfunction exists. Conversely, decreases in the glomerular filtration rate proportionally reduce the elimination of drugs or metabolites that are primarily excreted by the kidney.

Table 73-1. Drugs that Induce Hepatic Enzymes

Anticonvulsants	Nicotine
Barbiturates (short-acting)	Steroids
Tranquilizers	Rifampin
Ethanol—chronic usage	Spironolactone

Table 73-2. Causes of HBF Alterations

Decreased HBF	Increased HBF
Decreased arterial blood pressure	Chronic phenobarbital use
Decreased cardiac output	Increases in cardiac output
Increased venous pressure	
Hepatic hypoxia	
Cimetidine	
Alpha-agonist administration	
Controlled positive-pressure ventilation	
Positive end-expiratory pressure	
Halothane anesthesia (16% decrease)	
Halothane + non-intra-abdominal surgery (25% decrease)	
Halothane + intra-abdominal surgery (58% decrease)	
Spinal anesthesia (T7–T10) (19% decrease)	
Spinal anesthesia (T2–T3) (28% decrease)	

The characteristic of a drug that affects hepatic clearance most is a drug's hepatic extraction ratio, which is the amount of drug taken up by the liver in one pass proportional to the arterial concentration of that drug. Changes in HBF minimally affect the clearance of drugs with a low extraction ratio. On the other hand, changes in HBF greatly affect drugs that are extracted to a high degree. The opposite occurs with enzyme induction. Drugs that have a low extraction ratio undergo an increase in their extraction ratio when enzyme induction occurs. Therefore, highly extracted drugs are classified as blood flow–dependent, while those drugs with a low extraction ratio have enzyme-dependent kinetics (Table 73-3).

Pharmacologically-induced and hemodynamic aberrations are the most likely causes of changes in metabolism, although alterations in drug metabolism caused by genetic variation

Table 73-3. Drugs Classified by Hepatic Extraction Ratios

High Extraction	Intermediate	Low Extraction
Beta-blockers	Alfentanil	Amobarbital
Bupivacaine	Methohexital	Lorazepam
Fentanyl	Midazolam	Mepivacaine
Phenytoin	Vecuronium	Theophylline
Ketamine		Thiopental
Meperidine		Warfarin
Morphine		
Naloxone		
Pentazocine		
Sufentanil		
Lidocaine		
Isoproterenol		
Tricyclic antidepressants		

are more common than previously thought. The estimated prevalence of persons of European ancestry whose livers acetylate drugs rapidly is between 30 and 50 percent. For example, differences in acetylation rates probably account for the variance in fluoride levels seen in patients on isoniazid who are given isoflurane. In a more well-known disorder, approximately 1 out of 480 people are heterozygous for atypical pseudocholinesterase, while homozygotes occur in 1 of every 3200.

The second major category is changes in pharmacodynamics. Pathophysiologic alterations that increase anesthetic requirement include hyperthermia and hypernatremia. The minimum alveolar concentration (MAC) of halothane increases 8 percent for every 1°C increase in body temperature. Likewise, hypernatremia increases halothane requirements in dogs.

Drugs that increase central nervous system catecholamine levels generally increase the MAC of an anesthetic; however, other types of drugs may antagonize anesthetics. Patients using cigarettes, alcohol, or caffeine require more fentanyl to produce a desired result intraoperatively. Many other drugs reverse anesthesia in laboratory testing, but evidence indicates that they do not antagonize anesthetics clinically to a significant degree. A summary of antagonistic drugs is listed in Table 73-4.

Pathophysiologic conditions demonstrated to decrease anesthetic needs are severe hypoxia and hypercapnia. Beginning at a PaO_2 of 38 mm Hg, MAC decreases rapidly. Severe hypercapnia produces a similar result. MAC does not decrease until the arterial PCO_2 reaches 95 mm Hg. Likewise, cerebrospinal fluid pH has no effect on MAC until the pH drops to less than 7.1; MAC then decreases until complete narcosis occurs at a pH of 6.8. Perhaps because of a mechanism similar to that of severe hypoxia (decreased oxygen supply), significant hypotension (systolic arterial blood pressure < 40 mm Hg) also reduces the MAC of halothane.

Other abnormal conditions that decrease MAC include hypothermia (about 5% for every 1°C) and hyponatremia. Pregnancy and advanced age also diminish the requirements for both inhaled and local anesthetics. Halothane MAC is at its peak during infancy, while it reaches its nadir in the elderly. Mechanisms by which drugs reduce MAC include (1) depletion of central nervous system catecholamine levels (alpha-methyldopa) or inhibition of their release (clonidine), (2) blockade of sodium channels (verapamil, lidocaine), and (3) stimulation of *mu* opiate receptors (opioids). See Table 73-5 for a partial list of these drugs. Other drugs exert their action by less certain means.

Table 73-4. Drugs that Increase Anesthetic Requirements

Monoamine oxidase inhibitors	Tobacco?
Tricyclic antidepressants	Caffeine?
Cocaine—acute exposure	Cholinesterase inhibitors
Amphetamines—acute exposure	Steroids?
Chronic ethanol abuse	Naloxone?

Table 73-5. Drugs that Reduce Anesthetic Requirements

Alfentanil	Levodopa
Alcohol (acute administration)	Lidocaine
Alpha-methyldopa	Lithium
Amphetamines (chronic administration)	Morphine
Barbiturates	Nitrous oxide
Chlorpromazine	Pancuronium?
Clonidine	Scopolamine
Diazepam	Sufentanil
Fentanyl	Tetrahydrocannabinol
Hydroxyzine	Verapamil
Ketamine	

In summary, an essential part of the preoperative evaluation is to determine whether the anesthetist will encounter any factors that will change the patient's response to the anesthetic. Among the factors to be aware of are (1) medications that either induce or inhibit hepatic enzymes, (2) severe hepatic or renal failure, and (3) disease states and medications that reduce or increase the effect of the anesthetic. By carefully gleaning a patient's (or family) history of response to medications, the anesthetist may also be able to discern a genetic variation in the pathways of drug metabolism. Thus, by preparing for anticipated changes mishaps from either anesthetic overdose or underdose can be avoided.

SELECTED READING

Stoelting RK: *Pharmacology and Physiology in Anesthetic Practice.* Philadelphia: Lippincott, 1987. Pp 1–34.
Wood M: Pharmacokinetics for the anesthesiologist. *42nd Annual Refresher Course Lectures and Clinical Update Program.* American Society of Anesthesiologists. Lecture 244, pp 1–7.

74
Urticaria and Angioedema

DEFINITION

Urticaria, or hives, is defined as transient, erythematous wheals that affect the superficial layer of skin, usually associated with severe itching (pruritus). Angioedema is characterized by nonpitting edema that involves the deeper dermal layers and mucosal membranes; pruritus is absent, since sensory fibers are scarce in these tissues. Either disorder is considered acute if symptoms last less than 6 weeks and chronic if persisting longer than 6 weeks. Several different pathophysiologic mechanisms, with a wide variety of triggering agents, can culminate in urticaria or angioedema. These agents can be divided into two general categories, intrinsic or extrinsic, based on the source of the causative factor.

ETIOLOGY
I. Intrinsic
   A. Infection (hepatitis B, Epstein-Barr virus)
   B. Systemic disorders (connective tissue diseases, neoplasms)
   C. Psychogenic
   D. Hereditary angioneurotic edema
   E. Idiopathic
II. Extrinsic
   A. Drugs (penicillin, aspirin, sodium pentothal, *d*-tubocurarine)
   B. Foods (shellfish, nuts, eggs)
   C. Inhalants (pollen, animal dander)

D. Insect stings (hymenoptera)
E. Physical agents (mechanical, vibratory, thermal, solar, contact)

DISCUSSION

Initially, one should thoroughly review the patient's history and medication record. However, only 15 to 20 percent of all cases of chronic urticaria or angioedema are diagnosed in spite of the best medical efforts. In addition, it has been estimated that 20 percent of the population will have at least one episode of urticaria, angioedema, or both during their lifetime.

The patient may give a history of allergies to certain inhalants (pollen, ragweed), foods (shellfish, nuts, eggs), or insect stings. Episodes due to inhalants are usually associated with allergic rhinitis or bronchospasm; allergies to food or food additives are often more difficult to diagnose. A patient highly allergic to hymenoptera may require emergency intubation and resuscitation due to angioedema of the airway.

Other extrinsic causes of urticaria include drugs and physical agents. Current drug usage is not mandatory, since drugs taken as long as 1 month prior to the onset of symptoms may lead to hives with an associated serum sickness disorder; this delay may obscure diagnosis. The list of drugs that can produce hives is unlimited, since nearly all drugs have been associated with this disorder. The most common offenders, however, are penicillin and related antibiotics, aspirin, opiates, sulfonamides, and radiographic contrast media. Other drugs, such as sodium pentothal, morphine, and d-tubocurarine and its derivatives, can produce hives secondary to direct histamine release; in these cases, hives do not signify a true allergic reaction.

Physical agents can induce urticaria and account for about 15 percent of all cases. Dermatographism, a wheal and flare reaction following pressure to the skin, can be either immediate or delayed. Both cold and warm thermal stimuli may lead to urticaria; some conditions are acquired, while others are familial and transmitted as an autosomal dominant trait. Other miscellaneous categories include hereditary vibratory angioedema (autosomal dominant disorder characterized by angioedema following vibratory stimuli), solar urticaria (urticaria developing immediately after exposure to sunlight), and exercise-induced anaphylaxis (urticaria and angioedema immediately following exercise). Contact urticaria occurs when substances directly touch the skin. For example, hives have been noted in patients with myelomeningocele following contact with latex gloves; this sensitization is felt to develop secondary to chronic instrumentation of the bladder.

Certain intrinsic disease states can induce urticaria. Hepatitis B infections can produce immune-complex deposits in the skin, leading to urticaria. Cold urticaria can be acquired following Epstein-Barr virus infection. Urticaria may be a cutaneous manifestation of some systemic diseases (rheumatoid arthritis, lymphoma, leukemia, and systemic lupus erythematosus). Psychogenic factors can lead to a worsening of chronic urticaria.

Of all the intrinsic causes, the potentially most devastating is hereditary angioneurotic edema. It is an autosomal dominant disorder that may initially present as life-threatening airway obstruction. This condition is due to a deficiency of the enzyme C1 esterase inhibitor; in its absence, the complement cascade, once triggered, continues uncontrolled, leading to release of the mediators of anaphylaxis. Factors as minor as emotional stress may initiate the sequence.

SELECTED READING

Champion RH: A practical approach to urticarial syndromes: A dermatologist's view. *Clin Exp Allergy* 20 : 221, 1990.

75
Mydriasis

DEFINITION

Mydriasis is defined as the extreme dilation of a pupil. Pupil dilation is mediated by the sympathetic nervous system, while parasympathetic fibers cause constriction. Mydriasis may be either unilateral or bilateral.

ETIOLOGY

I. Unilateral
   A. Normal variant (anisocoria)
   B. Drugs (atropine, scopolamine)
   C. Uncal herniation
   D. Direct trauma to the globe
   E. Horner's syndrome
   F. Infections (uveitis)
   G. Adie's pupil
II. Bilateral
   A. Central nervous system pathology (brain death, midbrain lesions, deep coma)
   B. Drugs (cocaine, epinephrine)
   C. Light anesthesia

DISCUSSION

The first step is determining whether pupil dilation is unilateral or bilateral. Anisocoria, or inequality in pupil diameter, is a normal variant and the most common cause of unilateral dilation, occurring in 15 to 20 percent of the general population.

In these cases, the difference in pupil diameter should be less than 1.5 mm. Because of the condition's prevalence, the pupils should be evaluated prior to induction of general anesthesia.

Several other conditions produce unilateral pupil dilation. Drugs, primarily atropine or scopolamine, cause mydriasis by direct contact; usually the patient gets the drug on his fingers, as when applying a TransScop skin patch, then unknowingly rubs his eye. (In fact, this sequence happens so frequently that the package insert for TransScop patches warns patients to wash their hands thoroughly after handling.) Direct trauma to the globe can lead to disruption of the muscle apparatus that constricts the pupil. Uncal herniation of the temporal lobe, a terminal event from an expanding intracranial mass lesion, is associated with increased intracranial pressure or head trauma. Horner's syndrome causes the pupil on the affected side to be constricted, thereby causing the opposite pupil to appear dilated. Recent eye infections can lead to scarring and subsequent mydriasis. Adie's pupil is an abnormality of the myotonic reaction of the pupil. It usually appears in females in the third or fourth decade of life; patients complain of the sudden onset of blurry vision or notice that their pupils are unequal. It is due to disruption of the parasympathetic fibers but is without any clinical significance.

Bilateral mydriasis is due to either sympathetic stimulation or a central nervous system (CNS) lesion. Sympathetic stimulation, as occurs with light anesthesia or cocaine ingestion, can cause an increase in norepinephrine and subsequent pupillary dilation; in these cases, the pupillary light reflex is usually intact. CNS lesions, such as midbrain lesions, deep coma, or brain death, can produce dilated pupils that do not respond to light.

SELECTED READING

Roy FH: *Ocular Differential Diagnosis*, 4th ed. Philadelphia: Lea & Febiger, 1989. Pp 369–374.

76
Peripheral Edema

DEFINITION

Edema is defined as an increase in the interstitial component of the extracellular fluid compartment. The factors that determine fluid movement are referred to as the Starling forces and are related by the equation:

$$\text{Fluid accumulation} = K\,[(P_c - P_{if}) - \sigma(\pi_{pl} - \pi_{if})] - Q_{lymph}$$

Where K = permeability coefficient
     P_c = mean intracapillary (hydrostatic) pressure
     P_{if} = mean interstitial fluid pressure
     σ = reflection coefficient of macromolecules
     π_{pl} = oncotic pressure of plasma proteins
     π_{if} = oncotic pressure of interstitial fluid
     Q_{lymph} = lymphatic flow

The colloid oncotic pressure (COP) produced by the plasma proteins and the hydrostatic pressure within the interstitial compartment promote fluid movement into the vascular tree, while hydrostatic pressure in the vascular space and the COP in the interstitial fluid promote fluid movement into the interstitial space. Any fluid that leaks out of the vasculature is quickly removed by the lymphatic system. Of these five variables, the plasma COP, the intravascular hydrostatic pressure, and the lymphatic drainage are the major factors affecting fluid movement. Therefore, the causes of edema can be divided into three categories: (1) decreased plasma COP, (2) increased vascular hydrostatic pressure, and (3) impaired lymphatic drainage.

ETIOLOGY

I. Decreased plasma COP (hypoalbuminemia)
   A. Malnutrition
   B. Nephrotic syndrome
   C. Protein-losing enteropathy
   D. Severe hepatocellular disease
   E. Fluid overload (dilutional)
   F. Acute glomerulonephritis
II. Increased intravascular hydrostatic pressure
   A. Congestive heart failure
   B. Fluid overload
   C. Restrictive pericarditis (secondary to radiation, tumor)
   D. Impaired venous return (gravid uterus, thrombo-phlebitis, ascites, tumor)
III. Impaired lymphatic drainage
   A. Resection of regional lymph nodes
   B. Chronic lymphangitis
   C. Metastatic cancer

DISCUSSION

The first step in diagnosis is to determine whether the edema is localized or generalized. Localized edema usually indicates regional venous obstruction (thrombophlebitis) or lymphatic obstruction (following axillary node dissection for breast carcinoma). Once established, lymphedema may persist, since impaired lymphatic drainage leads to protein accumulation in the interstitium, which subsequently impedes the removal of retained fluid (increased π_{if}). Other causes of localized edema include inflammation and hypersensitivity, or may take special forms, such as ascites or hydrothorax.

Generalized edema is also referred to as pitting edema, since pressure on the area of fluid accumulation leads to a persistent indentation. It is in contrast to nonpitting edema (pretibial mxyedema), which is seen in Graves' disease. Generalized edema is secondary to either decreased COP or increased hydrostatic pressure. Since albumin is the major contributor to COP, absolute decreases due to increased losses (nephrotic syndrome, protein-losing enteropathy) or decreased production (malnutrition, severe liver disease) can lead to edema. Dilutional or relative hypoalbuminemia can be produced when large volumes of crystalloid solutions are administered intravenously. Whether relative or absolute, hypoalbuminemia leads to hypovolemia and subsequent salt and water retention, which exacerbates the hypoalbuminemia. Therefore, the albumin level decreases and the edema worsens. In early stages the fluid, although generalized, collects in the most dependent portion of the body due to gravitational forces (the ankles of standing individuals and the sacral area of supine patients); when total body edema develops, it is called anasarca ("dropsy").

The second pathologic mechanism is increased intravascular hydrostatic pressure. The most common cause is left ventricular dysfunction secondary to myocardial infarction, cardiomyopathies, and congestive heart failure. Increased hydrostatic pressure in the presence of normal left ventricular function can occur with restrictive pericarditis or with any condition that impairs venous drainage, such as thrombophlebitis or a gravid uterus.

Beneficial diagnostic studies include renal and hepatic function tests, urinalysis, and serum albumin levels. If these tests are normal, an echocardiogram can be obtained to evaluate left ventricular function. If restrictive pericarditis is suspected, it is best diagnosed using a pulmonary artery catheter to measure chamber pressures.

SELECTED READING

Epstein M: Disorders of sodium balance. In Stein JH (ed): *Internal Medicine*, 3rd ed. Boston: Little, Brown, 1990. Pp 844–853.

77
Increased Serum Enzymes

DEFINITION

Upon admission to the hospital, most patients have a variety of blood chemistries analyzed. Routine screening tests may reveal elevations in one or more values. Although occasionally these findings are insignificant, they frequently indicate an underlying pathologic process. Since no one enzyme is specific for one organ system or disease state, evaluating the patient and other laboratory studies will help elucidate the cause of the elevated value.

ETIOLOGY
I. Lactic dehydrogenase (LDH)
   A. Hemolysis (intravascular, traumatic venipuncture)
   B. Myocardial infarction
   C. Passive congestion of the liver
   D. Pulmonary embolism
   E. Rapidly proliferating tumors (lymphoma, leukemia)
   F. Hemorrhagic shock
II. Creatine kinase (CK)
   A. Myocardial infarction
   B. Skeletal muscle trauma
   C. Central nervous system (CNS) disorder (meningitis, cerebrovascular accident, hepatic coma)
   D. Duchenne's muscular dystrophy
III. Serum glutamic oxaloacetic transaminase (SGOT)
   A. Myocardial infarction
   B. Acute hepatocellular disease (hepatitis)

C. Skeletal muscle trauma
D. Other (chronic hypokalemia, acute pancreatitis)
IV. Alkaline phosphatase
   A. Obstructive liver disease
   B. Normal bone growth—children/adolescents
   C. Paget's disease
   D. Hyperparathyroidism
   E. Metastatic carcinoma to the bone

DISCUSSION

Lactic dehydrogenase (LDH) is actually a group of intracellular enzymes found in virtually all cells. Five different fractions, or isoenzymes, constitute the total LDH, with different concentrations of each isoenzyme found in different tissues. Elevation of the LDH indicates cellular damage, with the increase in a specific isoenzyme indicating the injured tissue. Probably the most common cause is hemolysis produced by a traumatic venipuncture. Intravascular hemolysis may occur for many reasons, including disseminated intravascular coagulation or a malfunctioning prosthetic heart valve. For reasons that are unclear, the LDH is increased in 60 to 80 percent of cases of pulmonary embolism. There may be a striking increase in LDH in patients with rapidly proliferating tumors such as lymphomas. Although present in hepatocytes, hepatocellular disease rarely leads to an increase in the LDH, although minimal elevations can occur with passive congestion of the liver.

The major concern is whether the elevation indicates myocardial cell necrosis. The LDH begins increasing at 24 to 48 hours post–myocardial infarction, peaking at 48 to 72 hours, and returning to normal by 10 days. Fractionating the enzymes in these cases is helpful; in a myocardial infarction, fraction 1 increases so that it exceeds fraction 2 (Fig. 77-1). These studies may be diagnostic when suspicious chest pain has occurred 3 to 5 days earlier.

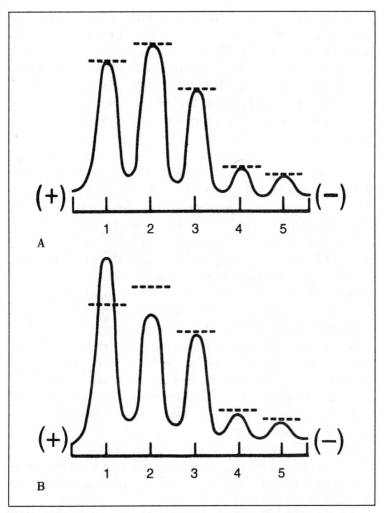

Figure 77-1. Representative LDH isoenzyme patterns with most frequent etiologies. A. Normal. B. Fraction 1 increased, with 1 becoming greater than 2: acute myocardial infarct. (From Ravel R: *Clinical Lab Medicine.* Chicago: Yearbook, 1978.)

The second serum enzyme is creatine kinase (CK). This enzyme has three isoenzymes, originating from the brain (CK-BB), myocardium (CK-MB), and skeletal muscle (CK-MM). Classifying the elevation according to the fraction will help distinguish skeletal muscle damage (intramuscular injections or trauma) from a myocardial infarction. The CK-MB fraction is the most sensitive laboratory indicator of myocardial damage. It rises 3 to 6 hours after the infarction, peaks at 12 to 24 hours, and returns to normal at 48 to 72 hours. However, a small percentage of skeletal muscle cells contain the CK-MB fraction; damage and regeneration of these cells, as occurs in the early stages of Duchenne's muscular dystrophy, may cause marked increases in this isoenzyme. This elevation does not indicate myocardial cell damage, in spite of the high frequency of cardiac disease in children with Duchenne's muscular dystrophy. The third fraction, CK-BB, is located primarily in neural tissues and may be increased in a wide variety of CNS disorders; elevation does not always occur and is not diagnostic of any specific CNS disorder.

Serum glutamic oxaloacetic transaminase (SGOT) is any enzyme located in the cells of the heart, liver, and skeletal muscle. In patients with myocardial infarctions, the SGOT becomes elevated at 8 to 12 hours, peaks at 24 to 48 hours, and falls to normal by 3 to 8 days. In patients with hepatocellular damage, such as acute hepatitis, the SGOT is markedly elevated and takes days to weeks to return to baseline. Other causes of elevations in SGOT include skeletal muscle damage (trauma, surgery), acute pancreatitis, and chronic hypokalemia.

The fourth enzyme, alkaline phosphatase, is found mainly in the liver and bones. It lines the biliary ducts and is an extremely sensitive marker to mild degrees of biliary obstruction; it may be elevated even when the total bilirubin is normal (see Chap. 28). With hepatocellular damage, the alkaline phosphatase is minimally elevated. The second source of this enzyme is the osteoblasts of bone. Elevations are normal in actively growing children and adolescents. However, in adults, they may indicate pathologic states such as hyper-parathyroidism, Paget's disease of bone, or metastatic carcinoma to the skeleton.

SELECTED READING

Griffiths J: Alkaline phosphatases: Newer concepts in isoenzymes and clinical applications. *Clin Lab Med* 9 : 717, 1989.

Lotts JA, Stang JM: Differential diagnosis of patients with abnormal serum creatine kinase isoenzymes. *Clin Lab Med* 9 : 627, 1989.

Wolf PL: Lactate dehydrogenase isoenzymes in myocardial disease. *Clin Lab Med* 9 : 655, 1989.

Index

Index

Page numbers in italics indicate figures; page numbers followed by t indicate tables.